Promoting Recovery in Mental Health Nursing

SAGE was founded in 1965 by Sara Miller McCune to support the dissemination of usable knowledge by publishing innovative and high-quality research and teaching content. Today, we publish over 900 journals, including those of more than 400 learned societies, more than 800 new books per year, and a growing range of library products including archives, data, case studies, reports, and video. SAGE remains majority-owned by our founder, and after Sara's lifetime will become owned by a charitable trust that secures our continued independence.

Los Angeles | London | New Delhi | Singapore | Washington DC | Melbourne

Promoting Recovery in Mental Health Nursing

Steve Trenoweth

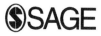

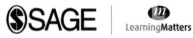

Learning Matters
An imprint of SAGE Publications Ltd
1 Oliver's Yard
55 City Road
London EC1Y 1SP

SAGE Publications Inc.
2455 Teller Road
Thousand Oaks, California 91320

SAGE Publications India Pvt Ltd
B 1/I 1 Mohan Cooperative Industrial Area
Mathura Road
New Delhi 110 044

SAGE Publications Asia-Pacific Pte Ltd
3 Church Street
#10-04 Samsung Hub
Singapore 049483

Editor: Alex Clabburn
Development editor: Richenda Milton-Daws
Production controller: Chris Marke
Project management: Swales & Willis Ltd,
Exeter, Devon
Marketing manager: Tamara Navaratnam
Cover design: Wendy Scott
Typeset by: C&M Digitals (P) Ltd, Chennai, India
Printed by CPI Group (UK) Ltd, Croydon, CR0 4YY

Library of Congress Control Number: 2016950575

British Library Cataloguing in Publication data

A catalogue record for this book is available from the
British Library

ISBN 978-1-4739-1304-2
ISBN 978-1-4739-1305-9 (pbk)

Contents

Transforming Nursing Practice is a series tailor-made for pre-registration student nurses. Each book in the series is:

- Affordable
- Mapped to the NMC Standards and Essential Skills Clusters
- Full of active learning features
- Focused on applying theory to practice

Each book addresses a core topic and they have been carefully developed to be simple to use, quick to read and written in clear language.

> An invaluable series of books that explicitly relates to the NMC standards. Each book cover a different topic that students need to explore in order to develop into a qualified nurse... I would recommend this series to all Pre-Registration nursing students whatever their field or year of study
>
> **Linda Robson**
> **Senior Lecturer, Edge Hill University**
>
> The set of books is an excellent resource for students. The series is small, easily portable and valuable. I use the whole set on a regular basis.
>
> **Fiona Davies**
> **Senior Nurse Lecturer, University of Derby**
>
> I recommend the SAGE/Learning Matters series to all my students as they are relevant and concise. Please keep up the good work.
>
> **Thomas Beary**
> **Senior Lecturer in Mental Health Nursing, University of Hertfordshire**

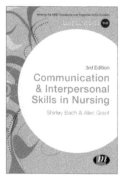

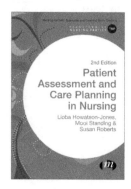

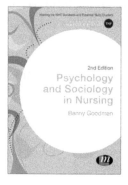

CORE KNOWLEDGE TITLES:

Becoming a Registered Nurse: Making the Transition to Practice
Communication and Interpersonal Skills in Nursing (3rd Ed)
Contexts of Contemporary Nursing (2nd Ed)
Getting into Nursing (2nd Ed)
Health Promotion and Public Health for Nursing Students (2nd Ed)
Introduction to Medicines Management in Nursing
Law and Professional Issues in Nursing (4th Ed)
Leadership, Management and Team Working in Nursing (2nd Ed)
Learning Skills for Nursing Students
Medicines Management in Children's Nursing
Microbiology and Infection Prevention and Control for Nursing Students
Nursing and Collaborative Practice (2nd Ed)
Nursing and Mental Health Care
Nursing in Partnership with Patients and Carers
Palliative and End of Life Care in Nursing
Passing Calculations Tests for Nursing Students (3rd Ed)
Pathophysiology and Pharmacology for Nursing Students
Patient Assessment and Care Planning in Nursing (2nd Ed)
Patient and Carer Participation in Nursing
Patient Safety and Managing Risk in Nursing
Psychology and Sociology in Nursing (2nd Ed)
Successful Practice Learning for Nursing Students (2nd Ed)
Understanding Ethics in Nursing Practice
Understanding Psychology for Nursing Students
Using Health Policy in Nursing
What is Nursing? Exploring Theory and Practice (3rd Ed)

PERSONAL AND PROFESSIONAL LEARNING SKILLS TITLES:

Clinical Judgement and Decision Making for Nursing Students (2nd Ed)
Critical Thinking and Writing for Nursing Students (3rd Ed)
Evidence-based Practice in Nursing (3rd Ed)
Information Skills for Nursing Students
Reflective Practice in Nursing (3rd Ed)
Succeeding in Essays, Exams & OSCEs for Nursing Students
Succeeding in Literature Reviews and Research Project Plans for Nursing Students (3rd Ed)
Successful Professional Portfolios for Nursing Students (2nd Ed)
Understanding Research for Nursing Students (3rd Ed)

MENTAL HEALTH NURSING TITLES:

Assessment and Decision Making in Mental Health Nursing
Critical Thinking and Reflection for Mental Health Nursing Students
Engagement and Therapeutic Communication in Mental Health Nursing
Medicines Management in Mental Health Nursing (2nd Ed)
Mental Health Law in Nursing
Physical Healthcare and Promotion in Mental Health Nursing
Promoting Recovery in Mental Health Nursing
Psychosocial Interventions in Mental Health Nursing

ADULT NURSING TITLES:

Acute and Critical Care in Adult Nursing (2nd Ed)
Caring for Older People in Nursing
Dementia Care in Nursing
Medicines Management in Adult Nursing
Nursing Adults with Long Term Conditions (2nd Ed)
Safeguarding Adults in Nursing Practice (2nd Ed)

You can find more information on each of these titles and our other learning resources at **www.sagepub.co.uk**. Many of these titles are also available in various e-book formats, please visit our website for more information.

Foreword

Sometimes revolutions are noisy and devastating, but sometimes they start quietly, in the places where people are subject to continual difficulty and distress. The recovery movement could be seen as just such a revolution. To say that successful implementation of the recovery model, in its original form, could transform services is not unreasonable; though there have been, and are, many challenges inherent in doing this. The tension that exists between the recovery approach and the continually dominant bio-medical model is not ignored in this book and it provides a balanced view of a complex subject. The book also goes some way to suggesting solutions to some of these challenges and suggests ways in which you, as nurses, can implement the model and support the approach in a way that will promote the likelihood of success. The book provides practical exercises that will help the reader to develop a stronger understanding of the recovery approach, the challenges of implementing it and opportunities to explore your own values and beliefs.

Much of the material in the first five chapters is usefully, and very powerfully, summarised in the last two chapters. Three key features of this book are, firstly, pointing out the power differential that exists in mental health care and the impact that this has on assisting service users to have control over their own lives, an essential element of the recovery process; secondly, the fundamental importance of nurses being human beings, exploring the common humanity of people and recognising that both staff and service users come up against mental distress during their lives, experiences that can be shared and explored to aid recovery; and thirdly, a call to action to the reader as a citizen of the community not just as a nurse to advocate for those in distress, to take a stand for equality and to discourage the co-option of the model to suit the needs of services rather than service users.

If you are a student nurse, a newly qualified nurse or even a nurse of some years standing looking for tips to update your portfolio of skills, this book will stand you in good stead for practice. It can be read as a whole but can also be dipped into section by section as you come across situations in practice, perhaps, that warrant further exploration of that particular subject. Engaging with this book will help you to become a more effective and safe practitioner of the art of mental health nursing, enhancing your ability to promote the recovery approach in health care and help those in mental distress to find renewed hope and personal power so they may once again live a life they feel is worth living.

Sandra Walker
Series Editor

About the editor and contributors

Editor

Steve Trenoweth has been a mental health nurse for 26 years. He has worked in a wide variety of mental health settings before entering higher education in 2003. He is currently a senior lecturer at Bournemouth University. He has authored several books, chapters and articles in nursing and health care, and is an editorial board member of the *British Journal of Mental Health Nursing*. He is a trustee of Project Nurture, a Dorset-based charity committed to enriching and enhancing the natural and built environment for those who are suffering from the effects of social exclusion and mental health difficulties.

Contributors

Wasiim Allymamod is a qualified nurse working in an acute service of a London mental health trust. He qualified from the University of West London with a first class honours degree in mental health nursing in 2008. His interests are cognitive behaviour therapy, positive health and mental wellbeing and psychosocial interventions.

Teresa Clark works for Certitude, a not-for-profit organisation that provides personalised support for people with learning disabilities, autism and mental health needs in London. She currently manages an employment, training and education service for Barnet, Enfield and Haringey Mental Health Trust's North London Forensic Service. The service was commissioned in response to the trust's acknowledgement that forensic patients require a personalised re-enablement approach to encourage and promote a successful transition into their communities. She is responsible for developing and facilitating an experts by experience programme within Chase Farm Hospital and a public involvement programme at the University of West London. The public involvement programme was created to assist the university to implement their public and carer involvement strategy through utilising members of the community who have had first-hand experience of the health care and mental health system to be involved in the training and development of their students. She is a trustee for Key Changes, a London-based charity that provides music engagement and recovery services in hospitals and the community for young people and adults experiencing mental health problems.

Sandra Connell qualified as a registered psychiatric nurse in Ireland in 2003, working for a short period in inpatient rehabilitation before moving into services in the community in Ireland. In 2010, Sandra registered with the NMC as a registered nurse in mental health; since moving to England Sandra has worked as a lecturer. She is a lecturer in mental health at Middlesex University and links with Barnet, Enfield and Haringey University Trust and is the service user educator co-ordinator for the mental health team at Middlesex University.

Sally Gomme currently works for West London Mental Health Trust and has also worked for many years in the voluntary sector. She has worked in project management and development but over the last twelve years has mainly taught and lectured in mental health with a focus on recovery and culture change. In her current role she is developing a Wellbeing Network in Hounslow, which has a non-clinical approach based on connecting people and strengthening communities.

Nicky Lambert is an associate professor at Middlesex University, where she is Director of Teaching and Learning for Mental Health, Social Work and Integrative Medicine. She is registered as a specialist practitioner (NMC) and is a senior teaching fellow with the HEA. She has a professional Twitter feed: https://twitter.com/niadla (@niadla) and is keen that all people with an interest in mental health engage together as a community to support good practice and challenge discrimination.

Phil Morgan is the lead for recovery and social inclusion for Dorset HealthCare University NHS Foundation Trust and co-lead for Dorset Wellbeing and Recovery Partnership, a partnership between Dorset HealthCare and the Dorset Mental Health Forum, which is a local peer-led third sector organisation. Phil is committed to exploring how recovery principles can shape our learning about ourselves, others and the organisations that we work within. Phil also works as a consultant for ImROC.

Rachel Perkins is senior consultant, Implementing Recovery through Organisational Change Programme (ImROC). She is also co-editor of the journal *Mental Health and Social Inclusion* and deputy chair of Equality and Human Rights Commission Disability Committee. In 2010 she was voted Mind Champion of the Year and awarded an OBE for services to mental health.

Helen Robson is a clinical nurse specialist for inpatient services within Berkshire Healthcare NHS Foundation Trust. She previously worked as a senior lecturer in mental health nursing at the University of West London for several years. She qualified as an RMN in 1992 and her clinical experience has been within both forensic mental health services and acute inpatient services.

Francis Thompson is a lecturer in mental health nursing, Faculty of Health and Social Work at the University of Plymouth. Francis has worked in a variety of clinical areas across inpatient and community services including older adults, the National Psychosis Unit and addictions services. He held a number of senior management roles in London where he focused on practice improvement and nursing education before moving into his current post as an associate professor of mental health nursing with Plymouth University.

Alison Tingle works part-time as the research development lead in the College of Nursing, Midwifery and Healthcare at the University of West London. In addition, Alison works part-time in the Policy Research Programme, a national research funding programme within the Department of Health's Science Research and Evidence Directorate. Her responsibilities include commissioning high quality, research-based evidence relevant to mental health to meet the needs of ministers, national policy makers and health and social care system partners.

Acknowledgements

I would like to thank Teresa Clark and particularly the service users at Certitude for their support of this project. Thanks also to Alex Clabburn and Richenda Milton-Daws at Sage for their patience and guidance.

We are grateful to service users from Certitude for supplying many of the voices heard across the chapters.

Thanks go to Dr Lioba Howatson-Jones for permission to base the case study in Chapter 2 (Ash and George, pages 23–4 of this book) on a case study ('Naeve's critical incident experience') in Chapter 10 of her book *Reflective Practice in Nursing* (3rd edition, Sage, 2016).

Introduction

Who is this book for?

This book is written primarily for mental health nursing students currently undertaking a pre-registration programme. However, it may also be of interest to qualified mental health nurses who wish to develop a deeper understanding of the recovery approach. In addition, those involved in the education of mental health nursing students, such as lecturers and clinical mentors, might find the book a useful resource for relevant teaching, learning and assessment activities.

Why *Promoting Recovery in Mental Health Nursing*?

Contemporary mental health care is an exciting, challenging and changing field. Established practices and traditional ways of understanding mental health and distress are being challenged, both by those who work within and those who use contemporary mental health services. The authority of mental health professionals and the legitimacy of their interventions are open to question as never before, and those who use mental health services are increasingly calling for greater involvement in how their experiences are understood and addressed.

In this changing and challenging environment, the roles that you will be required to perform as a qualified mental health nurse are becoming increasingly sophisticated. Not only will you be expected to identify, evaluate and apply various forms of information, research and evidence to your practice, but you will be expected to work in a recovery-focused and person-centred way with those who use mental health services and this will require an awareness of how your own assumptions, values and beliefs may affect your practice in both productive and non-productive ways. Contemporary mental health nursing therefore demands that you become an informed, self-aware and proactive mental health professional and central to achieving this is the ability to engage in critical thinking and critical reflection. This book will enable you to develop a deep understanding of how to promote the recovery approach in both the clinical and university setting and, importantly, it will allow you to consider the context of the debates, challenges and changes that characterise promoting this approach in contemporary mental health care.

Book structure

Chapter 1 asks the question, 'What is recovery?' It gives a contextual overview of the recovery approach, including policy and evidence, and how recovery can contribute to quality mental health nursing care. The concept of recovery will be defined, and in particular ideas of helping people to build a life which is meaningful to them; person-centredness; empowerment; choice; and taking responsibility and control for one's health. Traditional views of health will be contrasted with the contemporary view of recovery which will highlight individual pathways to recovery, including establishing personal goals, and contrasts will be made between clinical/medical and personal/social recovery.

Chapter 2 identifies the professional values, skills, knowledge and personal qualities needed by mental health nurses in order to work within the recovery approach, including working in partnership and collaborating with service users, an important aspect of contemporary mental health practice. There is also a discussion of how the mental health nurse should role model mentally healthy behaviour. The reader is offered advice and instruction on how to develop a helping relationship in order to support recovery-focused approaches, including maintaining hope, acting as role models for mental health, active listening, coaching, and how to engage and establish rapport.

Chapter 3 introduces the reader to the skills and knowledge that can be used to support an individual's recovery journey and to assist the individual to identify how their current experiences impact on their holistic and personal recovery. The chapter will clarify and reinforce the idea that recovery requires the active involvement of the service user. Supporting recovery within a multi-professional/multi-agency context will also be discussed. Concepts of empowerment, self-management, self-advocacy, control and agency, responsibility and personal recovery goals will be discussed. Options for treatment and care to support recovery, including medication, will be discussed along with the importance of user-defined treatment and intervention options.

Social inclusion is a vital component of recovery approaches. Chapter 4 explores the importance of supporting individuals in living, working and contributing to communities, undertaking valued social roles and forming social networks. The chapter will also consider the role of family, friends, carers and third sector organisations in the recovery process. Finally, it will look at culture, citizenship, stigma, work and employment.

Recovery approaches consider not only the challenges that a person may be facing in their lives, but also the skills and assets that help them to cope and manage their current troubles. In Chapter 5, we discuss the holistic concepts of positive health, skills, abilities, flourishing and mental/social capital and so forth. The reader can explore how people may be supported to develop a positive sense of self and satisfaction with life. This will include mental health and non-mental health resources, including peer support. In particular, we focus on how hope, optimism and resilience can influence mental wellbeing and satisfaction with life.

In Chapter 6, the authors consider how recovery can be promoted throughout the lifespan. In particular, the authors will consider recovery approaches with older people with dementia and for others towards the end of their lives. Chapter 7 pays particular attention to the challenges of utilising the principles and practice of the recovery approach in a variety of mental health care settings, including those where the service user may be compulsorily detained. Consideration will be given to recovery approaches in crisis intervention; early intervention; and in-patient, forensic, intensive care and community services.

Requirements for the NMC *Standards for Pre-registration Nursing Education*

The Nursing and Midwifery Council (NMC) has established standards of competence to be met by applicants to different parts of the register, and these are the standards it considers necessary for safe and effective practice. There are generic standards that all nursing students irrespective of their field must achieve, and field-specific standards relating to each field of nursing, i.e. mental health, children's, learning disability and adult nursing. This book uses those NMC standards, taken from *Standards for Pre-registration Nursing Education* (NMC, 2010), to help you understand and meet the competencies required for entry to the NMC register. In particular, the relevant standards of competence are presented at the start of each chapter so that you can clearly see which ones the chapter addresses. While most chapters have generic standards, you will also find that some chapters identify mental health field-specific standards.

Learning features

Throughout the book you will find activities in the text that will help you to make sense of, and learn about, the material being presented by the author.

Some activities ask you to reflect on aspects of practice, or your experience of it, or the people or situations you encounter. *Reflection* is an essential skill in nursing, and it helps you to understand the world around you and often to identify how things might be improved. Other activities will help you develop key skills, such as your ability to *think critically* about a topic in order to challenge received wisdom, or your ability to *research a topic and find appropriate information and evidence,* and to be able to make decisions using that evidence in situations that are often difficult and time-pressured. Finally, communication and working as part of a team are central to all nursing practice, and some activities will ask you to carry out *group activities* or think about your *communication skills* to help develop these.

All the activities require you to take a break from reading the text, think through the issues presented and carry out some independent study, possibly using the internet. Where appropriate, sample answers are presented at the end of each chapter, and these will help you to understand more fully your own reflections and independent study. Remember, academic study will always require independent work; attending lecturers will never be enough to be successful on your programme, and these activities will help to deepen your knowledge and understanding of the issues under scrutiny and give you practice at working on your own.

You might want to think about completing these activities as part of your personal development plan (PDP) or portfolio. After completing the activity, write it up in your PDP or portfolio in a section devoted to that particular skill, then look back over time to see how far you have developed. You can also do more of the activities if you identify a weakness in a key skill, and this will help build your skill and confidence in this area.

There are explanations in the Glossary for words in **bold** in the text.

Chapter 1
What is recovery?

Steve Trenoweth, Alison Tingle and Teresa Clark

NMC Standards for Pre-registration Nursing Education

Domain 1: Professional values

Field standard for competence

Mental health nurses must work with people of all ages using values-based mental health frameworks. They must use different methods of engaging people, and work in a way that promotes positive relationships focused on social inclusion, human rights and recovery, that is, a person's ability to live a self-directed life, with or without symptoms, that they believe is meaningful and satisfying.

Domain 2: Communication and interpersonal skills

4. All nurses must recognise when people are anxious or in distress and respond effectively, using therapeutic principles, to promote their wellbeing, manage personal safety and resolve conflict. They must use effective communication strategies and negotiation techniques to achieve best outcomes, respecting the dignity and human rights of all concerned. They must know when to consult a third party and how to make referrals for advocacy, mediation or arbitration.
5. All nurses must use therapeutic principles to engage, maintain and, where appropriate, disengage from professional caring relationships, and must always respect professional boundaries.
6. All nurses must take every opportunity to encourage health-promoting behaviour through education, role modelling and effective communication.

Domain 3: Nursing practice and decision-making

3. All nurses must carry out comprehensive, systematic nursing assessments that take account of relevant physical, social, cultural, psychological, spiritual, genetic and environmental factors, in partnership with service users and others through interaction, observation and measurement.
4. All nurses must ascertain and respond to the physical, social and psychological needs of people, groups and communities. They must then plan, deliver and evaluate safe, competent, person-centred care in partnership with them, paying special attention to changing health needs during different life stages, including progressive illness and death, loss and bereavement.

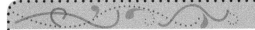

Essential Skills Clusters

Organisational aspects of care

10. People can trust the newly registered graduate nurse to deliver nursing interventions and evaluate their effectiveness against the agreed assessment and care plan.

Entry to the register

12. In partnership with the person, their carers and their families, makes a holistic, person centred and systematic assessment of physical, emotional, psychological, social, cultural and spiritual needs, including risk, and together, develops a comprehensive personalised plan of nursing care.

Chapter aims

After reading this chapter you should be able to:

- identify the key features of the 'recovery' approach and how it compares and contrasts to the biomedical model;
- describe how the recovery approach can contribute to quality of life for people with mental health problems;
- consider the implications of the approach for the delivery of mental health nursing care.

Introduction

This chapter gives an overview of the **recovery** approach, comparing and contrasting it to the **biomedical model** of mental ill-health, currently the most dominant paradigm of mental health care in England. We will also explore how mental health nurses can facilitate recovery and in particular how they can support people with mental health problems to build a life which is personally meaningful to them and to take control of their own health and wellbeing.

Recovery: the historical context

It is important to be able to place the recovery approach in a historical context in order to examine motivation for change, and to decide where to place it in a civil and human rights context. From the opening of the asylums to their closure in the 1960s and 1970s, followed by the move to community care in the 1990s, most people working within mental health services come to work to help people to get better, with genuine and passionate intent. This is the case whether their role is to design, manage or deliver these services. However, the containment and restrictive nature of these asylums limited the ability to form collective action and effectively prevented the growth of service user representation. In the 1970s, one organisation formed that can justifiably be called the originator of organised service user action, namely the Mental Patients' Union, with branches in various parts of the country (Campbell, 2005). In the mid-1980s, the service user movement began to gather pace with the rise of collective and individual advocacy across the country.

The recovery approach has developed from the growth of the service user movement which has carried an imperative for all mental health services to be humane, meet the needs and demands of the person and honour their human rights. Many individuals, such as Pat Deegan, have been inspirational in the development of this approach and take their place in service user history, particularly relating to the demand for change since the asylums. Judi Chamberlin's ground breaking book, *On Our Own*, first published in 1977, describes how people with mental health challenges can – individually and collectively, within and alongside wider communities – find solutions to the problems they face. The foundations of this work lay in the real-life narratives of people who had lived with and moved beyond the mental health challenges they faced, and have been developed and elaborated within this context (see O'Hagan, 2014).

Changes to service delivery have also, indirectly, catalysed the development of the recovery approach. For example, the 1980s strategy of providing care in the community and the closure of mental institutions was a catalyst for progressive collective communication and action. It was instrumental in the hugely significant service user organisation Survivors Speak Out that emerged throughout the 1980s, which was a key influence for further rights-based, user-led political and human rights organisations. The mental health charity Mind organised conferences which provided a fertile meeting ground for these ideas to flourish. The first of these, the 1985 Mind/World Federation of Mental Health Congress in Brighton, brought together national and international thinking (Campbell, 2005).

Recovery takes its place as an oppressed minority (i.e. mental health service users) seeks equality alongside other civil and human rights campaigns and follows the pathways of women's rights; rights of black and ethnic minorities; lesbian, gay, bisexual and transgender, and many more. It is important that we see recovery in its political and historical context lest we believe it is the benevolent gift of governments, mental health services or professionals. The right to recovery is a right demanded by the service user movement, and one to which everyone who needs it should have access.

Defining recovery

There are many definitions of recovery so it is useful to start with William Anthony's who, as Director of the Boston Center for Psychiatric Rehabilitation, developed a definition which is widely regarded today as important and valuable.

> *[A] deeply personal, unique process of changing one's attitudes, values, feelings, goals, skills and/or roles. It is a way of living a satisfying, hopeful, and contributing life even with*

limitations caused by the illness. Recovery involves the development of new meaning and purpose in one's life as one grows beyond the catastrophic effects of mental illness.
(Anthony, 1993)

This definition, along with many others, questions beliefs that began to be challenged in the 1980s and 1990s, namely, that mental illness was chronic and could only be contained and maintained. Many of these attitudes were still rooted in kindness and care, but held low expectations and a fundamental belief in illness and chronicity. The recovery approach rejects that notion and sees recovery as an expected outcome. It is personally defined and therefore will look very different for everyone, like all human growth. It can contain setbacks and is not defined by the use of services, the presence of diagnosis or the continued use of treatment. These can be absent or present in recovery.

Definitions of recovery recognise the impact of diagnosis and the subsequent journey of finding meaning in what has happened to the individual and discovering new sources of meaning and value. In this sense, recovery is

the lived or real life experience of people as they accept and overcome the challenge of disability. They experience themselves as recovering a new sense of self, and of purpose beyond the limits of disability.
(Deegan, 1988)

The recovery approach

The *recovery approach* stresses the holistic and biopsychosocial approaches while emphasising individual and personal pathways of recovery. It does not seek to denigrate the medical approach, but it places emphasis on the entire experience of the individual rather than a narrow frame of reference defined by a perceived illness. The recovery approach takes a different starting point to the medical model in that initial consideration is given to how the individual may be assisted to achieve a life which is personally fulfilling to them, recognising their strengths, assets and abilities, rather than focusing on disabilities, deficits and symptoms.

The recovery approach draws a distinction between **complete recovery** (in which an individual returns to their level of functioning before they experienced mental ill health often implying that the person has been 'cured' or *recovered*) and **social recovery** (which focuses on helping the person *towards* recovery, and involves an emphasis on social support, realistic planning, significant working relationships, encouragement, appropriate treatment, choice and self-management) (Warner, 1985; Matthews, 2008). In the latter case, much emphasis is placed on the ongoing process of *recover-ing* from mental health problems. Here, an emphasis is placed on supporting the person holistically with an aim to improve their overall quality of life despite the presence of 'psychiatric symptoms'. Hence, recovery in this sense

is not about regaining a problem-free life – whose life is? It is about living life more resourcefully, living a satisfying and contributing life, in spite of limitations caused by a continuing vulnerability to disabling distress.
(Watkins, 2001, p45)

Service user comment: What is recovery?

Recovery is a constant state for a service user. To begin with, recovery is something that you will work towards and once in that phase of your treatment it is ongoing. Reaching different levels, this can be judged by what you achieve while remaining settled in your core. Namely being symptom free. The only way I can describe this is, for example, a person who has used illegal drugs and attends an NA [Narcotics Anonymous] meeting. The core symptom of abusing the drug is gone; this is the start of recovery, however this person cannot be seen as cured. It's the steps. Support. Recognition. Acceptance. And ongoing supportive services received. These are the beginning stages of recovery. And just to note that a person can be 20 years clean and still an addict. This, I believe, is very similar to mental health. There is no cure, the medication only suppresses the illness and takes away the symptoms. It is up to the individual and supportive services to initiate recovery and recovery goals and for this to be constantly assessed, first and foremost by the service user depending on where they are in their recovery. And to work in conjunction with supportive services.

Practitioner comment: What is recovery?

Recovery is a very individual and personal journey. It isn't black and white and it's not as simple as 'getting better'. Within mental health, there are many factors which can aid this journey, and which can help to build the foundations to support the individual. Using recovery goals provides the individual with an opportunity to consider what they perceive to be important in their recovery at different times. These goals can be very diverse, depending on where that person is within their journey and where they want to get to. For some this might be to be discharged from hospital; to live independently; to be more active; to stop smoking; to get a job; to have a family, or to remain mentally stable.

Recovery is holistic. It is forever developing and is ongoing. As mental health professionals we can work with these individuals to help encourage them to always seek the best in themselves and to achieve their own personal goals.

The policy context

More contemporary perspectives of the recovery approach in England have been influenced by a guiding statement published in 2005 by the now defunct National Institute for Mental Health in England (NIMHE) (see Figure 1.1).

In 2008, the Centre for Mental Health published an influential and important document entitled *Making Recovery a Reality* (Shepherd et al., 2008). It provided indicators of how recovery can be promoted through practice in mental health settings, recognising the importance of a home, employment, a living wage and genuine control over one's life. It reinforced the need for services to be orientated towards hope and emphasised the need to build on an individual's strengths and abilities in the process of their recovery.

A broad vision of recovery [...] involves a process of changing one's orientation and behaviour from a negative focus on a troubling event, condition or circumstance to the positive restoration, rebuilding, reclaiming or taking control of one's life. Furthermore, a recovery-oriented system of care will:

- Focus on people rather than services.
- Monitor outcomes rather than performance.
- Emphasise strengths rather than deficits or dysfunction.
- Educate people who provide services, schools, employers, the media and the public to combat stigma.
- Foster collaboration between those who need support and those who support them as an alternative to coercion.
- Through enabling and supporting self-management, promote autonomy and, as a result, decrease the need for people to rely on formal service and professional supports.

Figure 1.1: Guiding Statement on Recovery (NIMHE, 2005)

In July 2009, the Future Vision Coalition (a group of UK-based charities and mental health organisations) set out a new vision for mental health. It argued for a broader, public health approach and saw that good mental health was important for an overall good quality of life. In this sense, mental health was an issue for everyone in society. It argued for effective positive mental health promotion to be a policy priority for the UK Government, including building resilience and targeted prevention work with at-risk groups.

A **person-centred approach** to care is embodied in health care policies, such as *Equity and Excellence: Liberating the NHS* (Department of Health (DH), 2010), the *NHS Constitution* (DH, 2013), the National Institute for Health and Care Excellence (NICE) pathway for *Patient Experience in Adult NHS Services* (NICE, 2012), the *Whole-Person Care* report (Royal College of Psychiatrists, 2013), and in mental health care terms, the strategy for England *No Health Without Mental Health* (DH, 2011). This strategy seeks to improve outcomes not only for people who have existing mental health problems but also to 'improve the mental health and wellbeing of the population and keep people well' (DH, 2011, p5). In this way, the current mental health strategy for England is as much about improving service delivery and the experience of care as it is about mental health promotion of individuals and communities:

If we are to build a healthier, more productive and fairer society in which we recognise difference, we have to build resilience, promote mental health and wellbeing, and challenge health inequalities. We need to prevent mental ill health, intervene early when it occurs, and improve the quality of life of people with mental health problems and their families.
(DH, 2011, pp6–7)

As implied by the title, *No Heath Without Mental Health* (DH, 2011) gives equal weight to mental and physical health, recognising that having a mental health problem increases the risk of long-term conditions (such as diabetes, respiratory and cardiovascular diseases) and early mortality. Furthermore, people who have chronic physical ill-health and painful debilitating conditions have an increased risk of developing mental health problems (Margereson and Trenoweth, 2010). The guiding values of the strategy are explicitly recovery-focused and person-centred, emphasising personalisation and control in helping people identify the outcomes, both physical and mental, that enable them to achieve a personally satisfying life (DH, 2011).

More recently, the Crisis Care Concordat (Department of Health and Concordat Signatories; DH, 2014), which was established to improve outcomes for people experiencing mental health crisis, has 'Promoting Recovery' as one of its four stages of the crisis care pathway.

Approaches to health and illness

Clinical recovery

> ### Activity 1.1   *Reflection*
>
> What does the term *recovery* mean to you? While you are reflecting on this, you may wish to take a few moments to think about and note down what is generally implied by the term *illness*.
>
> *You may wish to review your answers when you have finished reading the whole chapter.*

You might have said that *recovery* is an end-point – that is, the point when someone has actually *recovered* from an illness, perhaps when a person no longer has symptoms of an illness. In this way, recovery might mean that a person has been *cured* and this view of recovery is in keeping with the biomedical view of health and illness. This we have referred to in the book as *clinical recovery*.

Illness is often associated with perceptions of poor health resulting from disease – a state of being sick. Other words associated with the term can include sickness, impairment, disorder, ailment, affliction and so forth. You might have noted that the concept of *illness* implies a disease arising from a germ or infection, or a medical or biological problem associated with some form of bodily dysfunction. Applying this to the concept of mental health, we might assume that a *mental illness* has an underlying biological basis arising from some form of anatomical defect or physiological dysfunction within the brain.

There are two main systems which attempt to classify mental illnesses by assigning a diagnosis based on an assessment of symptom clusters: the World Health Organization's *International Classification of Diseases (ICD) 10th Edition* (WHO, 2007a) and the American Psychiatric Association's *Diagnostic and Statistical Manual of Mental Disorders (DSM) 5th Edition* (APA, 2013). When arriving at a psychiatric diagnosis, the psychiatrist seeks to make 'objective' judgements about a person's mental state before deciding which category of mental 'illness' (or 'illnesses') the person is suffering from.

There is some evidence which seems to suggest an underlying link between dysfunction of the brain and mental distress. For example, an excess of the neurotransmitter **dopamine** has been suggested as a precursor to **schizophrenia** and chronic depression and stress may lead to damage of the brain, particularly the **hippocampus**, **amygdala** and **frontal cortex** (Perna et al., 2003). Depression may also result from physical trauma to the brain leading to a disruption in the brain's ability to process information (Brown, 2004). Some degenerative brain diseases have clear organic aetiologies. In **Alzheimer's disease**, for example, neuroimaging reveals neural tangles in the brain which appear to kill brain cells. Poor nutrition and diet has also been linked to mental health problems and some nutrients such as folic acid, omega-3 fatty acids, selenium and tryptophan appear to reduce the symptoms of depression (Mental Health Foundation (MHF) 2006). Some infections, such as influenza, have been suggested to affect the development of the foetus resulting in an apparent increase of the risk of a diagnosis of schizophrenia in adulthood (Perna et al., 2003). There also appear to be heritability factors associated with many mental illnesses, with some studies suggesting that identical twins are three times more likely to develop schizophrenia if their twin also has this diagnosis, compared to non-identical twins (Kring et al., 2010).

Activity 1.2	*Research and evidence-based practice*

There are many medical treatments which are thought to help people experiencing mental distress. Commonly psychiatric medication is used for a wide variety of conditions. The National Institute for Health and Care Excellence (NICE) provides guidance on the effectiveness of treatments for particular conditions.

Visit the NICE website (**www.nice.org.uk**) and spend some time exploring NICE guidance on treatment choices for people with mental health problems.

Make notes on your findings. Does anything you have discovered surprise you? If so, you might want to discuss this with your mentor.

Holistic and biopsychosocial approaches to recovery

The biomedical model claims that biological factors (such as the anatomy and physiology of an individual's nervous system and their genetic make-up) are crucial risk factors in the development of a mental illness (Engel, 1977). However, Engel (1977) suggests that the role of biological predeterminants of mental distress may have been overemphasised. For example, assuming, for a moment, that there is clear medical agreement among those who make psychiatric diagnoses (Bentall (2003) suggests that there is not), some people point out that there is as yet no clear or definitive evidence to prove the connection between biological dysfunction and mental health problems (Bentall, 2003; Kring et al., 2010).

Others have suggested that a medicalised approach to mental disorder may impact adversely on an individual's recovery pathway. For example, there is potential danger in seeing a person solely in terms of their medical diagnosis – this process is known as **labelling**. Furthermore, authors such as Engel (1977) have argued that the medical model may be too reductive and subsequently may restrict our understanding of the complexity of health and illness. In particular, it may not understand how beliefs, expectations and hopes impact on the trajectory of recovery.

Activity 1.3 — *Critical thinking*

The World Health Organization (WHO) argued in 1946 that illness was 'not merely the absence of disease or infirmity'. In 2007, the WHO defined mental health as 'a state of well-being in which the individual realises his or her own abilities, can cope with the normal stresses of life, can work productively and fruitfully, and is able to make a contribution to his or her community' (WHO, 2007b).

What are the implications of the WHO's definition for our understanding of mental health and illness?

For individual service users?

For you as a nurse?

For the health care system?

You might like to discuss your responses with a colleague – have you identified similar things? If not, why might that be?

The WHO's definition of health and mental health takes a broad view, seeing it not simply as biological dysfunction, but also a reflection of our ability to function, cope within and make a contribution to society. This reflects the social nature of our functioning as human beings.

Concept summary: The biopsychosocial model

In 1977, Engel proposed a **biopsychosocial model** of illness. Here, Engel argued that there is a need to explore how psychological and social experiences combine with biological factors to affect the trajectory of illnesses. For example, how do discrimination, stigma and a lack of social inclusion affect an individual's health and wellbeing?

Engel argued that there is a need to include a broader view of the *person*, as well as the illness, to develop a more comprehensive understanding of their health problems.

Engel, G. (1977) The need for a new medical model. *Science*, 196, 129–36.

In 1977, Zubin and Spring argued for a 'new view of schizophrenia' which sought to explore how stressors could lead to a breakdown of coping in people vulnerable to schizophrenia. They assumed that people have a degree of vulnerability to schizophrenia which is *inborn* (for example, genetic and the 'internal environment' of the individual) and *acquired* (for example, the influence of traumas, perinatal complications and life events) which due to the interaction and presence of certain circumstances will challenge and provoke a crisis for a person's mental health. Such challenging circumstances (or 'exogenous stressors'), Zubin and Spring (1977) argue, include life events stresses (such as bereavements, marriage, divorce) which require a degree of coping and readjustment in the person's life. In vulnerable people, there may be a failure to cope and adapt to such stresses which may place their mental health under strain and increase the likelihood of mental ill-health or relapse.

A **holistic** view sees mental health as encompassing not only such social factors, but also physical, psychological, emotional and spiritual dimensions of self. As such, the model is an attempt to 'pool the wisdom from all of the models' (Zubin and Spring, 1977, p109). A holistic model has five interconnected dimensions (see Figure 1.2) (Swinton, 2001):

- Physical (the biological aspect of ourselves).
- Social (our relationships with others).
- Emotional (the way in which we feel about ourselves and our lives).
- Psychological (beliefs and perceptions that we hold about ourselves and others).
- Spiritual (the meaning that we attach to our lives).

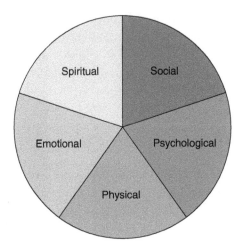

Figure 1.2: The holistic model

In this way, Swinton's model suggests that our experience of health and ill-health is likely to be multi-dimensional rather than one-dimensional. Importantly, as one dimension is affected this will impact on the other dimension of ourselves. This suggests that our physical, psychological and social and mental wellbeing are interrelated. For example, a problem with our physical health is likely to have implications for our social, emotional, psychological and spiritual wellbeing. 'Good' mental health, we may argue, can only result if each dimension is in harmony. That is, that we feel physically fit and able; that we make a valid and worthwhile contribution to the lives of others; that we feel positive about ourselves and our lives; that we hold ourselves in esteem and as a person of worth; and that we feel our lives have direction, purpose and meaning.

However, this would seem to imply that people with chronic or long-term conditions may not enjoy good mental health. This is clearly not the case as people who experience long-term physical and mental health issues do, of course, enjoy as good a quality of life as anyone.

However, it is also true that painful, debilitating and disabling health problems can impact significantly on quality of life, and pain and disability can undermine our subjective experiences of mental health and hence may lead to mental distress (Gureje, 2007).

People who subscribe to the biomedical model, however, do not inevitably rule out the interaction of biological factors with, for example, environmental experiences of an individual. Geneticists, for example, might argue that an individual has a *predisposition* to a particular illness but that environmental factors play an important role in whether this gene finds expression. Unquestionably, the medical model has offered much to people who experience mental distress and has helped many on their road to recovery and we would be wise not to dismiss this approach. However, the biomedical model tends to eclipse all others and holistic/biopsychosocial approaches remind us that there are other ways of understanding and supporting people who experience mental distress.

Within a holistic approach, then, medicine is one strategy to assist the person on the road to recovery and only helpful as far as it assists people to lead personally meaningful and satisfying lives. However, holistic/biopsychosocial approaches recognise there is equal value in promoting the psychological climate in the use of medication, and in having adequate discussion with people when medication is prescribed; acknowledging concerns about distressing side effects; and working actively with people to keep these to a level acceptable to the individual (MHF, 2012).

Personal views of recovery

The WHO definition of mental health described in Activity 1.3 recognises that we have a *sense* of our own mental health when we *realise* that our abilities help us to cope with the stresses of life, and that we can work productively and fruitfully, and make a contribution to our community (WHO, 2007b). That is, our own view of our own mental health is not something which can be assigned by others – it is a personal and 'subjective' experience. We are mentally healthy when we believe it; when we sense it; when we see ourselves behaving in mentally healthy ways. This, of course, has implications for the promotion of recovery from mental distress and implies that one is recovering when one *believes* that one is recovering.

Research summary: Belief in one's own recovery

Research (for example, Onken et al., 2002; Ralph, 2000; Ridgeway, 2001; Sells et al., 2006; Tooth et al., 2003) has identified a number of important factors which underpin an individual's personal view of their own recovery, including:

- self-determination;
- discovering a more active sense of self;
- valuing themselves as a person through their interactions with others;
- realisation of the need to help themselves and take responsibility for their distress;

- seeing the potential for richer identities other than that of a person with mental health problems;
- reflecting on positive experience leading to consideration of other potentials; exploring experiences with reference to current and possible self;
- finding ways to monitor and manage the symptoms of their distress;
- optimism and spirituality.

Leamy et al. (2011) undertook a systematic review of the recovery literature and they developed a conceptual framework of personal recovery based on five categories: connectedness, hope and optimism about the future, identity, meaning in life and empowerment.

However, where the biomedical approach dominates, the personal and subjective experience of the individual may not be emphasised save for the self-report of symptomatology. Take, for example, a person who reports 'hearing voices'. The biomedical approach would describe such a person as experiencing **auditory hallucinations** – an abnormal experience resulting from an underlying biological dysfunction which requires medical care and treatment. However, what if a person feels that such experiences do not significantly interfere otherwise with the quality of their life? What if the person does not see their experiences as abnormal? Would we require that they still receive medical care and treatment? Perhaps, as Barker (2004) suggests, consideration should be given to the significance of the experience for the individual:

> *If the person reports '500 fiddlers under his bed playing the Devil's music', we are interested to know the answers to two key questions: In what way this is a problem? What does this mean to him.*
> (Barker, 2004, p247)

Service user comment: A personal view of 'recovery'

As a long-term service user living successfully back into the community, I am greatly encouraged with any attempts that move away from the medical model of recovery. Ever since the 1959 Mental Health Act, patients have been seen as their diagnosis and 'labelled' as such, rather than being seen as a human being with problems and distress. For service users we see our recovery as starting from the first day of going into hospital and that it doesn't really stop. The holistic approach with more service user involvement in their care and therapy is fundamental to achieve a good recovery outcome. Coupled with good support and supervision once the individual is back in the community. Again it is important to emphasise the need for service involvement in their care, 'Therapy should be done with us, not to us'. It is important for the service user to have some 'ownership of their progress'. The importance of staff training and support is key to recovery.

In this personal view, the service user is sharing their experiences of the impact of the medical model and the stigma that this may bring. They argue for a more inclusive approach, where health care staff and service users can work together to support the person on the road to their own personal recovery.

Recovery and evidence-based practice

In modern health care, emphasis is placed on health care interventions which are based on 'sound' evidence and those that lead to positive clinical outcomes are favoured. Indeed, the role of the National Institute for Health and Care Excellence (NICE) is to systematically review and appraise 'best available' research evidence, assessing the quality of such evidence in terms of its clinical and cost effectiveness. Evidence is then interpreted before advice (in the form of 'clinical guidelines') is issued to guide health care practice. Health care professionals are involved in the clinical guideline development (CGD) process as well as a range of individuals from differing backgrounds, including members of the public who have an interest in the topic area. Emphasis is placed on the integrity of the findings and any member who has a vested or commercial interest (such as those who have links to pharmaceutical companies) must declare this.

The quality of evidence which is used to inform the CGD process is based on a hierarchy as shown in Table 1.1.

Grade	Type of evidence
Ia	Evidence from a meta-analysis of randomised controlled trials
Ib	Evidence from at least one randomised controlled trial
IIa	Evidence from at least one controlled study without randomisation
IIb	Evidence from at least one other type of quasi-experimental study
III	Evidence from observational studies
IV	Evidence from expert committee reports or experts

Table 1.1: Hierarchy of evidence used by NICE

From this, clinical recommendations are graded as shown in Table 1.2.

Grade	Evidence
A	Directly based on Category I evidence
B	Directly based on Category II evidence or extrapolated from Category I evidence
C	Directly based on Category III evidence or extrapolated from Category I or II evidence
D	Directly based on Category IV evidence or extrapolated from Category I, II or III evidence

Table 1.2: Grading of recommendation by NICE

Grades of evidence: Which is best?

It might be assumed that Grade I or II evidence is the best form of evidence and must be applied to an individual who is experiencing mental distress. For example, the NICE guidelines for depression in adults (NICE, 2009), based on systematic reviews of research findings, recommend the use of antidepressants and cognitive behavioural therapy for people experiencing moderate symptoms of depression. This is the best available evidence from studies involving large populations and gives an important indication of what might work best for most people. However, we must also be aware that within a recovery-focused approach, and in working collaboratively with people, we need to support people in deciding care and treatment options based on their own individual preferences and wishes that would best help them to achieve a personally satisfying life. This may mean that the person rejects what is recommended by NICE preferring to opt for treatments, such as complementary and alternative therapies, as they believe that this would work better for them in achieving their personal goals.

Of course, if we are experiencing ill-health, we will want care and treatment which is the most effective way that we can be supported to resolve our current troubles and difficulties. Furthermore, the duty of care of any health care professional is to offer care and treatment which is most likely to improve a personal's health and wellbeing. NICE guidelines support this as they are based on an extensive review of relevant research. Research that is favoured by the NICE guidelines (that is, Grade I and II evidence) tends to come from studies where there has been some degree of control taken over measuring or manipulating **variables**. The ultimate aim of such studies is to demonstrate the effect of a variable (or variables) on another (or others).

However, NICE guidelines are biased towards research from large population studies using variables which are amenable to study and which often have clear and measurable outcomes (such as the abatement of particular symptoms or the ability of a person to return to a previous level of functioning). From a recovery model perspective however, research findings from a large *population* study may not be desirable, wanted or helpful to all *individuals* from within that given population. Furthermore, complex and subjective phenomena (such as the personal experience of recovery or mental health and wellbeing) may not be amenable to measurement or randomisation. Research which may illuminate personal recovery journeys, for example, might use different methodologies, such as qualitative or mixed-method studies. Such approaches often reveal rich information which clarifies complex phenomena, and provide holistic insights into personal experiences. However, such approaches often use small sample sizes and lack control of variables, and may therefore be considered lower quality evidence and may not inform NICE's clinical guidelines (see Tables 1.1 and 1.2). This potentially poses a significant challenge to the adoption of recovery-focused research in mental health care.

In person-centred, recovery-focused care, the starting point is not necessarily the population within which the person is located (and which population would this be in any case: Gender? Race and ethnicity? Diagnosis?) but with the individual and what is acceptable and helpful to them in supporting a life which is personally satisfying and meaningful. While this does not preclude consideration of the 'evidence' in supporting and promoting a person's recovery, the choices that a person makes in deciding which is most helpful to them is likely to be more complex, and may involve biopsychosocial and holistic factors resulting from an individual's personal and individual experience.

Service user comment

When it comes to recovery, it means many different things to different people. The best you can do is to be mindful of the values at the beginning of this chapter, and encourage each individual to find a path they want to take of their own volition with support and encouragement of course. But there will be a thousand paths they don't want to take before they find one they do, and they should be encouraged to find their own holistic notion of recovery, not as is often the case, encouraged to do what others might think is good for them. Of course you're going to get people who want to, for better or worse, do their own thing and be belligerent when it comes to the input of services. But equally you can only do your best to encourage independent proactivity and at least you'll know you did what you could for the best of any given individual. Remember, recovery is about helping make someone's life as full and productive as it can be and helping them chose what that means to them, and eventually setting them free! And helping them should they require assistance again.

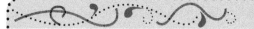 Chapter summary

In this chapter, we have given an overview of the recovery approach and contrasted it with the biomedical model of mental ill-health. We have heard from service users who welcome the approach as being a positive contribution in assisting them to achieve a personally defined quality of life.

However, no amount of treatment or therapy can 'cure' the stereotypes, prejudice and social discrimination that so limit the growth and potential of individuals. Neither can they 'cure' poverty, poor housing, unemployment and isolation: these are social, political and human rights issues and require us to engage with a broader agenda.

This chapter has highlighted three important things about what the recovery approach stands for:

- Recovery is situated in the context of the person's life – not that services will fix someone or make them 'better' but repositions health services as something that can be part of the support someone participates in to enable them to 'live well.'
- Recovery enables people to integrate their experience of mental health problems into their own life, so that it does not become about 'getting rid' of something but trying to understand the experience, find some meaning and live as well as possible.

- Recovery promotes different forms of knowledge, especially understanding the lived experience of a health condition and the idea that people and communities can have their own solutions. Through valuing the lived experience of someone with mental health problems or a health condition it enables us to take into account their experience of stigma, discrimination, and their cultural, social and economic reality.

Further reading

Bentall, R. (2003) *Madness explained: Psychosis and human nature.* London: Penguin.

An important book, if rather complex at times, which argues against a purely medical understanding of mental ill-health. Bentall argues that mental illness 'labels' such as schizophrenia are meaningless and criticises the medical approach to mental health care.

Useful websites

www.mentalhealth.org.uk/a-to-z/r/recovery Mental Health Foundation.

www.signpostuk.org/recovery/recovery-model Signpost UK.

www.rethink.org/living-with-mental-illness/recovery Rethink Mental Illness.

www.mentalhealthcare.org.uk/recovery Mental Health Care.

www.centreformentalhealth.org.uk/recovery Centre for Mental Health.

Chapter 2
The mental health nurse and recovery

Francis Thompson

NMC Standards for Pre-registration Nursing Education

Domain 1: Professional values

1. All nurses must practise confidence according to *The Code: Standards of conduct, performance and ethics for nurses and midwives* (NMC, 2015), and within other recognised ethical and legal frameworks. They must be able to recognise and address ethical challenges relating to people's choices and decision-making about their care, and act within the law to help them and their families and carers find acceptable solutions.

4.1. Mental health nurses must work with people in a way that values, respects and explores the meaning of their individual lived experiences of mental health problems, to provide person-centred and recovery-focused practice.

8.1. Mental health nurses must have and value an awareness of their own mental health and wellbeing. They must also engage in reflection and supervision to explore the emotional impact on self of working in mental health; how personal values, beliefs and emotions impact on practice and how their own practice aligns with mental health legislation, policy and values-based frameworks.

Domain 2: Communication and interpersonal skills

1. All nurses must build partnerships and therapeutic relationships through safe, effective and non-discriminatory communication. They must take account of individual differences, capabilities and needs.

5. All nurses must use therapeutic principles to engage, maintain and, where appropriate, disengage from professional caring relationships, and must always respect professional boundaries.

Domain 3: Nursing practice and decision-making

5.1. Mental health nurses must work to promote mental health, help prevent mental health problems in at-risk groups, and enhance the health and wellbeing of people with mental health problems.

8.1. Mental health nurses must practise in a way that promotes the self-determination and expertise of people with mental health problems, using a range of approaches and tools that aid wellness and recovery and enable self-care and self-management.

Domain 4: Leadership, management and team working

4. All nurses must be self-aware and recognise how their own values, principles and assumptions may affect their practice. They must maintain their own personal and professional development, learning from experience, through supervision, feedback, reflection and evaluation.

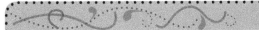

Essential Skills Clusters

Care, compassion and communication

1. As partners in the care process, people can trust a newly registered graduate nurse to provide collaborative care based on the highest standards, knowledge and competence.

3. People can trust the newly registered graduate nurse to respect them as individuals and strive to help them to preserve their dignity at all times.

5. People can trust the newly registered graduate nurse to engage with them in a warm, sensitive and compassionate way.

6. People can trust the newly registered graduate nurse to engage therapeutically and actively listen to their needs and concerns, responding using skills that are helpful, providing information that is clear, accurate, meaningful and free from jargon.

Organisational aspects of care

9. People can trust the newly registered graduate nurse to treat them as partners and work with them to make a holistic and systematic assessment of their needs; to develop a personalised plan that is based on mutual understanding and respect for their individual situation promoting health and well-being, minimising risk of harm and promoting their safety at all times.

Chapter aims

After reading this chapter you should be able to:

*   describe some of the values which underpin helping relationships;
*   understand some of the professional and policy frameworks which underpin the values-based practice within which nurses must operate;
*   have an understanding of how organisational values and the working environment can affect the nurse's ability to enact their personal and professional values and promote recovery;
*   have an understanding of how values and interpersonal skills can enhance or detract from your ability to form effective therapeutic relationships to promote recovery.

Introduction

This chapter explores the values, skills and personal qualities needed by mental health nurses to work effectively in a person-centred, recovery-orientated way. It outlines how our values as mental health nurses underpin effective engagement with service users to promote recovery. This includes a focus on developing a helping relationship to support recovery-focused approaches. The chapter also discusses how nurses can maintain positive person-centred approaches while under personal and organisational pressure.

Recovery and the mental health nurse

Mental health nurses are the largest group of people working with service users and have the potential to make a major contribution to the health and welfare of people with mental health needs (Cowman et al., 2001; Cleary, 2004; DH, 2006a). In 2006, the chief nursing officer's (CNO) review of mental health nursing, *From Values to Action* (DH, 2006), stressed the need for mental health nurses to address the holistic needs of service users, in an evidential and supportive way. Furthermore, nurses should be able to respond meaningfully and collaboratively to the complex physical and mental health care needs and wants of the service user group in a modern health care context (DH, 2006b).

Many authors have described the core qualities of the mental health nurse which may facilitate recovery-focused care. Certainly, a sense of patient-centred, caring concern is one of the most important resources nurses bring to care (Cowman et al., 2001; Barker and Buchanan-Barker, 2005). Caring is, according to Olsen (1997, p516), 'not part of treatment, it is the reason for treatment. Caring is, then, the very essence of nursing.' Nurses often have cited the importance of skills which are commensurate with the recovery approach. For example, in a study by Peck and Norman (1999), interpersonal skills were seen to be highly valued by nurses themselves, such as the skills of attentive listening, complex skills of reassuring, instilling confidence, and enabling and facilitating patients' goals. The ability to sustain relationships with people over time, and to relate to different people at different levels whilst working towards goals, were also seen to be important. Nurses in this study felt that general requirements were a positive outlook on life, energy and enthusiasm for life, faith in patients' capacity to change and an ability to instil hope. Furthermore, acceptance, seeing good and bad in people and the ability to maintain boundaries and contain and deal positively with fear, anxiety and anger, and human qualities, such as compassion, integrity, honesty, reliability, kindness, concern and patience, were crucial to nursing care (Peck and Norman, 1999).

In 1999, Barker et al. undertook a qualitative study which sought to define the core activities of mental health nurses and again highlighted the apparent complexity of the role. Nurses need to be several things at different times depending on context or circumstances. At times, nurses expressed a need to be ordinary and human (characterised by the depth and quality of time spent with service users and the depth of knowledge gained between nurse and service user). Indeed, 'the trick of being ordinary' emerged as a key unique skill in another study and 'Relating to patients in an "ordinary" person-to-person way emerged as central to the nurses' role' (Peck and

Norman, 1999). At other times, the need to be 'professional' (characterised by the exercising of professional judgements for and on behalf of service users) was identified. However, a key activity was that of being an intermediary or translator:

> *Translation emphasised the nurse's need to be multi-lingual: conversing easily with professional colleagues, in the language of psychiatry; yet able to speak to with people and their families, in ordinary parlance.*
> (Barker et al., 1999, p280)

The ability of the mental health nurse to work collaboratively and in partnership is vital. This involves listening to service users' expertise, and by providing consistent and reliable support through meaningful dialogue. As Watkins (2001) put it:

> *More than anything else they need to engage in a dialogue with practitioners to reach some kind of shared definition of their situation and what should be done about it [by] developing a dialogue in which people can uncover the problems of living they face; discover the meaning of the disabling distress and begin the process of recovery.*
> (Watkins, 2001, p46)

However, while technical and professional skills are important, it seems that the service users find the personal qualities of mental health professionals equally important in supporting their recovery (Mental Health Foundation (MHF), 2012).

There are many ways in which mental health nurses can support and promote a recovery approach in their practice. Certainly, a person-centred approach, which recognises that people may follow their own personal pathway to recovery, is essential. The role of the nurse must be collaborative, supportive and informative, helping people to confidently manage their own health care needs wherever possible, and knowing how much support the person may need at times. The nurse should be hopeful and optimistic, understanding the individual's strengths and assets as well as limitations. The person with mental health problems should be enabled to make their own choices and the nurse will need to be able to promote safety at the same time as enabling positive risk taking. The nurse will need to be able to work collaboratively with significant others in the service user's life, be they friends, family members, other health care professionals and advocates. And finally, nurses must be aware of the balance between promoting autonomy, and other factors such as staff relationships, organisational processes and issues of power which may undermine recovery-orientated approaches.

Case study

Ash is a third-year mental health nursing student on placement in a mental health secure unit. One young patient, George, had been sectioned and admitted after smashing up the family home and a stand-off with police. He had been off work with severe stress for a couple of weeks immediately beforehand.

(continued)

continued . . .

His family had found the experience of his outburst extremely traumatic and were reluctant to visit him, although his sister had been enquiring after him regularly.

Ash could see that George was withdrawn and did not speak much, so every day he was on duty, he spent some time sitting with him and trying to draw him out. By the second week George was starting to mumble some responses. By the third week Ash managed to coax him to come downstairs for his lunch.

A couple of days later, George's sister, Sarah, came to visit. George asked for Ash to be present when they met. George and Sarah met in the common room. At first everything appeared to be going well, but then George lost his temper when Sarah asked him where he would go after leaving the unit because he could not go back home. Ash ushered Sarah out of the room and returned to George. Although he felt anxious, Ash was able to maintain a calm exterior which gradually helped George to calm down. Ash's mentor had been observing his communication interactions over this period of time and was very impressed with Ash's handling of this volatile situation.

Professional values and personal qualities

Our values, beliefs and assumptions make us who we are; they develop throughout our lives and often go unnoticed. We often simply don't question them as they are so integral a part of us. However, these parts of our character are absolutely critical to our ability to engage with and work effectively with other people.

A **personal value** as defined by the *Oxford English Dictionary* is:

Principles or standards of behaviour; one's judgement of what is important in life.

Activity 2.1	Reflection

Take a moment to reflect on the following questions:

- What is a personal value?
- Are professional values different to these?
- Can you identify some of your core values and beliefs and how might your values influence the way you work with people?

If possible, discuss your thoughts with a fellow student.

Values underpin our behaviour in a given situation and there are a number of frameworks outlining the values deemed to be necessary to work as a mental health nurse. The Nursing and Midwifery

Council (NMC) (NMC, 2015) in *The Code* sets out the professional standards and behaviours required for registration as a nurse. They fall under four main categories:

- Prioritise people.
- Practise effectively.
- Preserve safety.
- Promote professionalism and trust.

Page 1 of *The Code* (NMC, 2015) highlights the importance of these principles and values:

> *While you can interpret the values and principles set out in the Code in a range of different practice settings, they are not negotiable or discretionary.*

In other words, nurses must act in a way that is consistent with *The Code* in order to remain registered as nurses.

The Department of Health (2015) also sets out a number of explicit values in the NHS Constitution. Users of services funded and provided by the NHS have a right to expect that these will be upheld. Professionals will:

- Work together in the best interest of patients.
- Treat all patients with respect and maintain their dignity.
- Be committed to quality of care.
- Show compassion.
- Work to improve lives.
- Remember that everyone counts.

In 2012 the chief nursing officer (CNO) for England, Jane Cummings, outlined what she saw as the values fundamental to nursing which she coined as the '6C's': Care, Compassion, Competence, Communication, Courage and Commitment. The NMC (2010, p22) also outlines some specific standards relating to values and recovery-orientated practice in the standards for competence:

> *Mental health nurses must work with people of all ages using values-based mental health frameworks. They must use different methods of engaging people, and work in a way that promotes positive relationships focused on social inclusion, human rights and recovery, that is, a person's ability to live a self-directed life, with or without symptoms, that they believe is meaningful and satisfying.*

There must be a link between our own beliefs and values, the values of health service(s) and the values required by our professional organisation, the NMC, and as mental health nurses it is important that we continually reflect on our values and respect the values of others.

Activity 2.2   *Critical thinking*

Look up and read *The Code* (NMC, 2015); ask a colleague to read *From Values to Action* (DH, 2006b). Once you have read these consider and discuss:

- Are there any values in these documents that you disagree with or would struggle to enact?
- Can you think of a situation from practice where you or others may not have demonstrated these core values and what did or should you have done about it?
- Do you think it is possible to work effectively as a mental health nurse if you do not share the values set out in these documents?

Caring: values underpinning developing therapeutic relationships and promoting recovery

The **therapeutic relationship** is at the heart of effective nursing care (Peplau, 1952; Rogers, 1956; Egan, 2010). A therapeutic relationship is one in which the primary focus is the service user, the aim of which is to enable collaborative working to support recovery. This approach starts with the person, not the disease or diagnosis. The key to effectively supporting people in their recovery is about the rebuilding of a person's life, hopes, dreams and aspirations and not just about the alleviation of symptoms, important though this may be (Deegan, 2007). Key to this is developing a strong trusting relationship (Forchuk and Reynolds, 2001). Watkins (2009, p177) reminds us that:

> *[Caring] is more about being than doing ... a basic philosophy, rather than a technique, which involves being with people in a way that creates the conditions for growth and change.*

Caring is at the heart of effective relationship building and respecting the person you are working with underpins this. Egan (1994) felt that respect means 'prizing people simply because they are human' (p51) and for Watkins (2009) nurses must demonstrate this through valuing the person's views and experiences.

Nursing, medicine and the role of the nurse in promoting recovery

Historically, there has been a split between what is sometimes termed *psychiatric nursing* and that of *mental health nursing* (Barker and Buchanan-Barker, 2011). This was largely played out in the 1990s but continues today (see, for example, Barker and Buchanan-Barker, 2011). The term *psychiatric nursing* is seen to be grounded in the 'medical model of psychiatric diagnosis and containment of abnormal behaviour' which Barker and Buchanan-Barker (2011) see as paternalistic and controlling. *Mental health nursing* on the other hand represents a values-based, person-centred and recovery-focused approach (Cahill, 2009; Forchuk and Reynolds, 2001). Barker and Buchanan-Barker (2011) argue that nurses in the UK still tend to operate in a framework of bio-medicine, an overarching paradigm which they argue is based on 'misplaced compassion' and, at times, coercion. Barker and Buchanan-Barker's position seems to be that the medical model may be at odds with recovery as the inherent system of 'diagnose and treat' imposes a way of thinking about people which does not inherently take into account their needs and wishes. 'Misplaced compassion' could be described as the desire of nurses to help the people they are working with and may therefore be trapped within this frame of reference; seeing care through the lens of 'treating' conditions rather than working with and respecting people's view and beliefs to enable recovery.

This perceived split described by Barker and Buchanan-Barker (2011) may also have a bearing on the nurse's ability to remain resilient and enact the values that underpin effective working with people. Perhaps working in a team where nurses (and other health care professionals, carers and service users) do not have a shared view of the causes or mechanisms of development of mental health problems; the way to 'treat' or support people with these conditions can lead to conflict and disagreement. Such differences in health professionals' fundamental beliefs, as outlined by Barker and Buchanan-Barker (2011), could lead to difficulties for individual nurses (and patients) in working environments which may in turn exacerbate stress and burnout. For example, Leiter and Maslach (2009) in their study into burnout in 677 Canadian nurses demonstrated that sharing values with colleagues played a key role in protecting nurses from feeling emotionally exhausted and depersonalised when under pressure at work.

Few people, however, would argue that mental health problems are purely rooted in one's biology or that interventions other than medicines have no value; as outlined in Chapter 1 there is a good deal of evidence which supports the use of medicines and this approach to 'treating' mental health conditions. Similarly, few people would argue against the concept of working with service users in partnership. The recovery approach is, of course, not necessarily at odds with the biomedical model and good practice in all approaches stresses collaborative decision-making and promoting choice (e.g. NMC, 2010, 2015; DOH, 2008, 2011). However, we may argue that the recovery approach emphasises the importance of supporting and maximising the patient's independence and choice and in compassionately and skilfully focusing on personal meaning for the individual, their desires, strengths and abilities. In the recovery approach, the focus is on listening and engaging with others; in supporting people through conversation to understand their own frame of reference and goals and in crafting plans with people which they enact to support them living their lives in the way they want to.

The quality of a therapeutic relationship seems to have considerable value in supporting an individual's recovery. Lambert and Barley (2002) argue that only 15% of the outcome in therapy is due to the modality of therapy with 40% due to 'extratherapeutic' change (change that would occur without any formal therapy input), 15% service user expectation and 30% common factors (in particular the therapeutic relationship). This lends itself to the conclusion that what have been termed non-specific therapeutic or 'common' factors (supportive relation-ships, person-centred approaches, values and listening skills) may have more of an influence on treatment outcomes than the mode of therapy itself and supports Rogers' (1956) assertion that personal attributes and values may be all that are required for therapeutic change to take place (see Chapter 3: Supporting recovery).

Demonstrating values: key concepts in team working and communication

In order to provide effective care, we should seek to work with, understand and engage peo-ple using mental health services and also other staff we are working with who may not share our own point of view. Paying attention to the way we communicate as nurses is critical in the formation of positive working relationships with colleagues. Our colleagues have their own personal history, hopes, fears, dreams and aspirations. In a recovery approach, our aim should be to support people to connect with and maximise their own skills and resources to promote their wellbeing regardless of whether they have come to us for help and support, or if they are our colleagues. Also remember that you are a person, as everyone, with your own hopes, dreams, aspirations and beliefs which will have an impact on the relationship; you are not just a 'professional' and should not assume that you are right or that you are just there to give advice or 'make' the person better. Working effectively with people in mental health services requires the recognition of traditional power dynamics not only in the nurse–patient relationship but also amongst those we work with, lead and manage. Egan (2010) highlights the need to meet people as equals, acknowledge the resources of others as well as our own, share power, make the process participative rather than directive and share our knowledge to support people's self-efficacy.

Enacting values in practice

In recent years the recovery movement has gained ground and publications such as *Refocusing the Care Programme Approach* (DH, 2008) and *The Code* (NMC, 2015) emphasise the need to have an increased focus on personalised care through better engaging service users. This chapter has discussed the importance of values-based practice and the professional and national policy doc-uments which support and require us to deliver person-centred compassionate care. However, Logan et al. (2011) point out that despite much clinical guidance emphasising the importance of service user participation and choice, practice standards are inconsistent. Cameron et al. (2005) argue that mental health nurses' interactions with service users are often not 'therapeu-tic'. Other authors also point to a lack of evidence of engagement and participation happening in practice (Langan and Lindow, 2004; Better Regulation Commission, 2006; Leitner and Barr, 2011). Timmermans and Mauck (2005) argue that while standards and guidelines are in theory supportive to practice, they do not, in general, lead to changes in the practice of health care professionals. These concerns are brought into focus by a number of recent national issues: the shocking abuse of vulnerable patients in 2011 at Winterbourne View described by the DH (2012), and the failings at the Mid Staffordshire NHS Foundation Trust (Francis, 2013) have led to widespread criticism about health care delivery.

Activity 2.3   *Research and evidence-based practice*

Look up and read the executive summary of the final report of the *Mid Staffordshire NHS Foundation Trust Public Inquiry* (2013) also known as the Francis Report. You will find it at: **http://webarchive.nationalarchives.gov.uk/20150407084003/http://www.midstaffspublic inquiry.com/report**

Then, read the summary of *Transforming Care: A National Response to Winterbourne View Hospital* (DH, 2012), available at: **www.gov.uk/government/uploads/system/uploads/ attachment_data/file/213215/final-report.pdf**

Consider:

- What do you think might some of the reasons be for practice failings and lack of engagement with people who used these services? How could you ensure you continue to give excellent and compassionate practice when under pressure?
- Have you seen examples where people were not enacting the values of the NMC *Code* or the NHS Constitution in practice?
- Look up and read your placement provider's incident reporting and 'whistleblowing' policies and discuss with a colleague: what actions would you take if you came across poor practice; would you feel supported in doing this?

Personal and professional values underpin good nursing practice, and undoubtedly an ability to enact the values of the health service and the nursing profession can lead to care failures (Francis, 2013). Sully and Dallas (2005) point out, however, that organisations, professions and groups develop shared accepted norms which influence and govern the way that people in that organisation behave. Traynor (2014) argues that we need to take a broader view of the causes of poor care delivery: poor leadership, lack of staff and other resources, and use these to help nurses to build an understanding of the impact that working under pressure can have on their ability to enact their values in practice. The culture and structure of the working environment and support available to the nurse may play a more important role in an individual's behaviour than simply the person's character traits and personal values.

Traynor's (2014) conclusions are broadly supported by findings in the literature such as those from Van Bogaert et al. (2013) who found that practice environments were predictive of nurses' assessments of the quality of care delivery. The environment in which you are working has a substantial influence on your practice; an influence which you need to be aware of, reflect on and take steps to ensure you are resilient enough to stand by your values, recognise where you need to challenge practice and seek the support you need to be an effective, compassionate, recovery-orientated nurse.

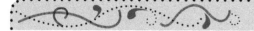

Chapter summary

Mental health nurses need to be aware of the fact that the values and structure of the organisations they work in can have an effect on the way they practice. They need to reflect on and be mindful of this and, at times, courageous enough to challenge poor practice and environments and cultures in which poor practice can grow and flourish. Nurses must work within the values and principles set out by the NMC and in various national mandates and need to find a way to build these values and principles into their practice. Values and beliefs can only be demonstrated to others through behaviour and how nurses behave will either promote or inhibit the people who we care for in their recovery. Enacting these values in the way we communicate is essential if we are to support people to achieve their goals.

Further reading

Barker, P. and Buchanan-Barker, P. (2011) Myth of mental health nursing and the challenge of recovery. *International Journal of Mental Health Nursing*, 20: 337–44.

Department of Health (2012) *Transforming care: A national response to Winterbourne View Hospital.* London: Department of Health.

Francis R. (Chair) (2013) *Report of the Mid Staffordshire NHS Foundation Trust Public Inquiry.* London: The Stationery Office.

Nursing and Midwifery Council (2015) *The Code: Professional standards of practice and behaviour for nurses and midwives.* Available at: www.nmc.org.uk/globalassets/sitedocuments/nmc-publications/revised-new-nmc-code.pdf

Traynor, M. (2014) Caring after Francis: Moral failure in nursing reconsidered. *Journal of Research in Nursing*, 19 (7–8): 546–56.

Watkins, P. (2009) *Compassionate care: A guide for mental health practitioners.* London: Elsevier.

Useful websites/resources

www.england.nhs.uk/wp-content/uploads/2013/12/MH6Cs.pdf Department of Health.

www.gov.uk/government/policies/mental-health-service-reform Mental Health Service Reform.

www.england.nhs.uk/wp-content/uploads/2016/02/Mental-Health-Taskforce-FYFV-final.pdf The Five Year Forward View of Mental Health.

Chapter 3
Supporting recovery

Helen Robson, Sally Gomme and Francis Thompson

NMC Standards for Pre-registration Nursing Education

Domain 1: Professional values

3.1. Mental health nurses must promote mental health and wellbeing, while challenging the inequalities and discrimination that may arise from or contribute to mental health problems.

4.1. Mental health nurses must work with people in a way that values, respects and explores the meaning of their individual lived experiences of mental health problems, to provide person-centred and recovery-focused practice.

Domain 2: Communication and interpersonal skills

1.1. Mental health nurses must use skills of relationship-building and communication to engage with and support people distressed by hearing voices, experiencing distressing thoughts or experiencing other perceptual problems.

5.1. Mental health nurses must use their personal qualities, experiences and interpersonal skills to develop and maintain therapeutic, recovery-focused relationships with people and therapeutic groups. They must be aware of their own mental health, and know when to share aspects of their own life to inspire hope while maintaining professional boundaries.

6.1. Mental health nurses must foster helpful and enabling relationships with families, carers and other people important to the person experiencing mental health problems. They must use communication skills that enable psychosocial education, problem-solving and other interventions to help people cope and to safeguard those who are vulnerable.

Domain 3: Nursing practice and decision-making

7. All nurses must be able to recognise and interpret signs of normal and deteriorating mental and physical health and respond promptly to maintain or improve the health and comfort of the service user, acting to keep them and others safe.

7.1. Mental health nurses must provide support and therapeutic interventions for people experiencing critical and acute mental health problems. They must recognise the health and social factors that can contribute to crisis and relapse and use skills in early intervention, crisis resolution and relapse management in a way that ensures safety and security and promotes recovery.

Domain 4: Leadership, management and team working

3. All nurses must be able to identify priorities and manage time and resources effectively to ensure the quality of care is maintained or enhanced.

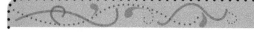

Essential Skills Clusters

Care, compassion and communication

1. As partners in the care process, people can trust a newly registered graduate nurse to provide collaborative care based on the highest standards, knowledge and competence.

2. People can trust the newly registered graduate nurse to engage in person-centred care empowering people to make choices about how their needs are met when they are unable to meet them for themselves.

3. People can trust the newly registered graduate nurse to respect them as individuals and strive to help them to preserve their dignity at all times.

6. People can trust the newly registered graduate nurse to engage therapeutically and actively listen to their needs and concerns, responding using skills that are helpful, providing information that is clear, accurate, meaningful and free from jargon.

Organisational aspects of care

18. People can trust the newly registered graduate nurse to enhance the safety of service users and identify and actively manage risk and uncertainty in relation to people, the environment, self and others.

By the first progression point:

18.3. Under supervision assesses risk within current sphere of knowledge and competence.

By the second progression point:

18.8. Under supervision works safely within the community setting taking account of local policies, for example, lone worker policy.

Chapter aims

After reading this chapter you should be able to:

*   identify the barriers to developing recovery-focused therapeutic relationships, including resistance to change;
*   consider the ways of supporting people to develop personal recovery strategies;
*   describe the process for structuring recovery conversations;
*   consider how hope and optimism are related to a person's recovery;
*   listen to recovery narratives and personal stories.

Introduction

Supporting recovery requires a considered understanding of the recovery approach, and a commitment to recovery values and objectives. There can be many assumptions about this and a wide variety of understandings, so it is an important element of good recovery practice that a common recovery value base is shared within teams. It can be the case that the word 'recovery' is often used without first agreeing its meaning, or checking that all those participating in the dialogue have the same understanding. If we are to support recovery in mental health, we need to begin by establishing exactly what we mean by the word 'recovery' and checking that all involved parties understand the term in the same way. We also need to identify any perceived barriers to the idea of recovery, and whether service users, families or professionals are in any way resistant to this goal.

The focus on clinical recovery, as opposed to personal recovery, within mental health services may be seen to support the 'treatment' of people in order to reduce 'risky behaviours'. This is in stark contrast to the philosophy of personal recovery. The recovery approach stresses the importance of the individual feeling that he or she is in control of their own health care experiences. Service users must feel that they are directing the care that is being planned in collaboration with the mental health care team, and be confident that they are in control of decisions about prioritising need and planning appropriate steps to enable their recovery goals to be achieved. It is also important to be aware that not all of a service user's goals or needs might, on the face of it, appear to be mental health focused. If a goal is of significant value to that individual, however, then it is likely to benefit his or her wellbeing and result in a positive impact for that person (Keeling and McQuarrie, 2014).

In this chapter we look at the various ways in which mental health nurses can develop their practice to support personal recovery and to enable collaborative care, and how nurses may attempt to overcome the challenges to recovery-focused practice.

Delivering recovery-focused nursing care

The overall aim of nursing care is to ensure that service users have the necessary support, information, resources, skills and networks to manage their own personal recovery and to help and enable them in identifying and securing the necessary resources to achieve this. The nurse may be viewed as a guide or facilitator of this process, offering the opportunity for the service user to identify what is important to them, in the short term as well as in the longer term and beyond their illness (Matthews, 2008).

Carl Rogers developed the concept of person-centred therapy in the 1950s. He proposed that there should be an underlying assumption that the nurse (or therapist) is not trying to direct the service user. Rather, he argued, their role is one of supporting the service user to explore what is happening and to provide an environment in which that individual can develop in a way that creates positive change. He continued by suggesting that change happens within therapeutic relationships and he described the 'core conditions' which are essential if any therapeutic change is to occur:

- Genuineness and transparency (congruency).
- Unconditional positive regard.
- Empathy.
- Warmth and being non-judgemental.

If these conditions exist and, importantly, if they are effectively communicated to and experienced by the service user, and continue over a period of time, then constructive change will occur. Nothing else is required to enable this change (Rogers, 1956/1962).

Miller and Rollnick (1991) developed an engagement and counselling technique called motivational interviewing. They developed this from the concept that the way in which a person is spoken to can either enhance or minimise engagement and motivation to change. Motivational interviewing attempts to explore a person's uncertainty and ambivalence about making changes to their lives. It is guided by the idea that motion to change should not be imposed from without in the form of arguments from the nurse, but rather needs to be elicited from within the person. Motivational interviewing supports the idea that nurses should work alongside service users to elicit their desires and support self-efficacy in making changes to their lives. In a similar vein, Schien (2013) argues that we should focus on asking rather than telling; he terms this 'humble enquiry'. The essential thrust of Schien's argument is that we need to know the things that others know in order to do our jobs and that to do so we need to ask questions respectfully with an awareness that different people come from differing points of view.

Thurgood (2009) argues that the values of the health care professional will have a significant impact on engagement. Thurgood cites the following as being central to the worker:

- being needs-led and service user centred;
- being flexible, responsive and creative;
- maintaining optimism and hope, perseverance, patience and realism;
- negotiation and seeing the service user as expert;
- advocacy;
- being willing to take positive risks, promoting choice and sharing information;
- being culturally sensitive;
- being honest, genuine, trustworthy and respectful.

Ackerman and Hilsenroth (2003) examined the factors which promote engagement and a positive therapeutic alliance. Their review found attributes such as openness, interest, flexibility, trustworthiness, warmth and honesty had a positive influence on effective relationship building.

In developing a recovery-focused relationship, the nurse will need to help identify with the person their own personal strengths and reflect with them on their ability to solve their own problems from previous experience (Slade, 2009a). Personal resilience is enhanced by the experience of others expressing a belief in that person and their ability to meet the challenges they face. In this regard, a relationship which is focused on hope and the respectful regard for the person's lived experience is essential.

Activity 3.1   *Critical thinking*

Think of an interaction you have witnessed, for example on a recent clinical placement, between an experienced mental health professional and a service user.

- Did there appear to be a bond of trust between the professional and the service user?
- Did you feel the encounter was a positive one?
- How has it impacted upon your view of how you would like to conduct such an encounter?

In the light of your response to this interaction, and in the context of the paragraphs above, how easy do you find the idea of involving a service user in decisions about how their care is managed?

You might want to discuss your feelings with a colleague, always maintaining confidentiality if you are talking about encounters with or between other people.

Service user comment: The value of mutual respect

God. It was all about God … how powerful and controlling He is … how totally Evil He is. These concepts of God explained my experience of life at that time. They explained why earthquakes and floods were claiming hundreds of lives. They explained why war was tearing people apart. They explained why cancer and the panoply of illnesses that kill human beings existed. They explained why murders, rapes, all terrible crimes, took place. They explained human suffering. My suffering.

And my suffering was great – I felt the pain of humanity in my heart – but there was absolutely nothing I could do about it. I was powerless in God's Evil working of reality. This made me angry, very angry with God. So I struggled. I tried to gain some kind of control in my life. But what could I do?

I cut myself. I threw up what I ate to lose weight – a lot of weight. I poisoned myself by taking too much medication. And I didn't die … somehow the fact that I was not being 'harmed' by my actions made me INVINCIBLE. No matter what God did to me in my life He could not make me feel any lower than this, so in a funny sort of way I had a tiny morsel of control. Then God got in my head. He started talking to me. God was playing with power when He made His commands. It was terrifying. And it was humiliating …

Psychiatrists tried to make my life more bearable and safe. They started by 'commanding' me to take anti-psychotic medication; threatening that if I didn't take it they would take me into hospital and 'force' me to take the medication. Again, I obeyed. Sleep. Sleep. And more sleep. Deathly tired. No longer able to think, let alone work. My head was just empty … at least God had stopped talking.

And it was at this point, when God was silent, that my recovery story began. I was introduced to a remarkable community psychiatric nurse (CPN) who spent several years engaging with me. She listened. I listened. We had a mutual respect for our thoughts and beliefs. And of course, mutual respect can only rise when

(continued)

(continued)

each person shares something to be respected. My CPN shared some of her cultural background (Nigerian) and described beliefs held by many in Nigeria about spiritual matters. She encouraged me to see that I was not the only person in the world who considered themselves to have had 'knowledge' revealed to them by a Divine or spiritual Being; nor was I the only person to have attributed negative power to such a Being. She never judged me or anyone else as being right or wrong. Instead she helped me accept there are other thoughts out there, some akin to mine in certain aspects. And helped me realise that I am not so alone.

Once we were past the initial 'certainty of knowledge' that I deemed my thoughts to be, once we started working with my thoughts, my CPN gently challenged me to think more about them. She encouraged me to apply the logic I had used to justify the thoughts originally to test them again and see if they could withstand the scrutiny. Gradually I had to admit, conceptually and rationally, that my thoughts were not knowledge, but belief. I still have internal wrangling with this idea – I believe my thoughts are knowledge and truth, but as a thinker I HAVE to concede that I cannot know this, only believe it.

This work, years of work, took me to a place in my head where I could benefit from cognitive behaviour therapy and subsequently mindfulness training. Both of which have strengthened me in my fight to gain control and power. For the space of the last four years I was given the gift of another amazing CPN – again, a woman who listened, who shared, meaning I wanted to listen and to share. In the therapeutic relationships I had with both these women I trusted them implicitly. Their kindness and the bond our rapport established led me to care deeply about them. I believe they cared about me. I still do care but our paths have moved apart – location changes, promotions, moving on …

The problems I've described started in 1997. Having had support since then from family, the community mental health team and therapy teams in dealing with a diagnosis of schizophrenia and what it entails brings me to now, when I am developing a modicum of power in my battle with schizophrenia:

I work.

I have friends.

I'm in a long-term relationship.

I've been discharged into 'shared care'.

And I CHOOSE to have an anti-psychotic depot injection every two weeks – it helps me keep God on the periphery of my world.

It helps me live my life.

Author comment: The value of mutual respect

This narrative by a service user encapsulates her experience of both her illness, and the distress and suffering she experienced whilst acutely unwell. It is clear from the account that these initial contacts involved a perceived lack of personal control and implicit threats when faced with information about treatment.

> *Although the outcome has been very positive, one can't help postulate over the quality of the overall experience, and how this might have been very different had this lady benefited from the same respectful, sharing relationships she had with her two community psychiatric nurses from the outset. It is clear from her story that she was very distressed at this time and in need of understanding and help. The prescription for medication was a catalyst for change, but what this lady has really valued, and has been pivotal in her recovery story, is the depth of engagement and mutual respect that was integral to the relationship she developed with the two CPNs. There was a real sense of sharing and partnership that she valued, and a commitment in terms of time and investment in their relationship which was essential to the recovery process. The skill of the two CPNs in offering an opportunity for her to make some personal sense out of what she was experiencing and in contextualising these experiences undoubtedly supported her in retaking personal control and making the life choices which have led her to her recovery story.*

Listening to recovery narratives and personal stories

There will be a set of circumstances and a story that led a person to be where he/she is now. We tell ourselves stories which describe and explain our lives, allowing us to make sense of what we have experienced and what we are experiencing. Over time people's stories shift and change to accommodate changes in their lives. Allowing people to tell their story, or a part of their story (when they want to), can allow them to make sense of themselves in new and different ways. This can be a catalyst for change in itself, as well as a way of building hope, future goals and developing plans to achieve them.

Nurses do well to try working with service users in order to create a shared understanding of the set of circumstances that have led to their situation and the factors that may be maintaining it. This allows the service user to clarify both their own understanding and their hopes and ambitions; it allows you both to understand what the person's difficulties are at this moment, and to explore their strengths, resources and aspirations which they need to build on and develop for the future. It allows you to set up clear, agreed plans for how to proceed based on a mutual understanding of the situation. Your job is to set up a relationship to enable a dialogue to take place which supports the person to feel in control and able to trust you and be confident that you will not judge them. You need to be genuinely interested and attentive, you need to listen and you need to set up the conversation in a way which maximises the chances of this happening. This is the role of the nurse and it is skilled and intense work but it can also be a joy and is a privilege.

Effective communication to support relationship building

We all possess the ability to listen; the key part is being interested. We must be attentive and reflective enough as a nurse to develop interest in the people we are working with, even the ones who don't share our values and beliefs, or who we find difficult to relate to. In supporting recovery, there are a number of skills to pay attention to which will maximise your ability to engage and communicate but being and demonstrating the following are vital to doing this well: a non-judgemental attitude, empathy, genuine curiosity and paying attention to the person (Rogers, 1956/1962; Barker and Buchanan-Barker, 2005).

Activity 3.2   *Communication*

It is best to try this activity with three fellow students or colleagues.

Divide into pairs. The individuals in each pair must take 2–3 minutes to tell the other person something interesting and unusual about themselves. For example, something you remember from your primary school days, or a quirky anecdote involving a hobby. (It should be something your colleagues won't already know but also something you don't mind sharing.)

Now swap partners. You need to pass on the story you have just heard to your partner in the new pair. Listen to each other carefully.

Next, swap partners again so that the person who has heard the 'passed on' story can re-tell it to the person who originated it.

Finally, all meet together as one group and share your findings. How well did the stories travel? How far did you recognise your own story in the form it came back to you? What have you learned about your listening skills from this activity?

Relationship building starts from the first time you meet the person you are working with. Beck (2011) outlines the following areas to concentrate on to maximise engagement:

- Good fundamental skills in communication and setting up conversations to enable accurate understanding of the service user's issues.

- Sharing your understanding of the situation.

- Collaborative decision-making.

- Seeking feedback from service users.

- Adapting your approach to the individual.

- Supporting people to solve their own problems to reduce distress.

Activity 3.3   *Reflection*

Reflect upon a really positive encounter you had with another person you did not know very well. This does not need to be an encounter in a professional context, but it should be one that left you feeling good about yourself and about the other person.

Jot down a few things you remember about the encounter. Think about body language, eye contact, whether one of you spoke much more than the other, whether you felt affirmed, appreciated or judged.

Some suggestions about what you might have experienced are given at the end of this chapter. They may not mirror your feelings exactly but they will give you some idea of what might make an encounter really positive for another person.

Structuring recovery conversations

General 'chit chat' or 'phatic' communication is important in developing therapeutic relationships and is often overlooked (Morrisey and Callaghan, 2011). Don't be afraid to just have 'normal' conversations with people you are working with but the emphasis should be on being a friendly professional and not a professional friend. For more formal therapeutic discussions it is useful to set up conversations in a more structured way to emphasise that this is a more purposeful session, and the table below outlines some basic steps which are useful to consider; you will need to use the skills outlined above throughout this process.

Process	Considerations
Preparation	*Self awareness* – Consider how you are feeling; will this impact on the conversation? Take a moment to prepare yourself. What are your goals and intentions? Have you thought of things from the service user's perspective? Are you clear about what you think you want to achieve from the meeting? Remember that this meeting is for the service user's benefit not yours. What might they want to achieve? How will you find out what this is? Attending to this is often the main thrust of the conversation.
	How will you be able to maintain interest, positive regard for the person, empathy and warmth? This is especially important if you are struggling to engage with the person or you are anxious about the conversation or need to discuss problems the person is having with behaviour or discuss issues of conflict with boundaries. In such cases it may be useful to review the person's history to reframe your thinking about their circumstances and behaviour.
	The person you are about to speak to – What do you know about them? Are there any likely issues with engagement, safety, culture or language barriers? Do you need an interpreter or some support for the conversation? How do you feel about the person? It is important that you reflect on these issues to enable you to anticipate any potential pitfalls and risks.
	The environment – Is the environment conducive to the conversation? Will you or the service user be distracted? Is it safe? Have you allowed enough time for the meeting?

(continued)

Table 3.1 (continued)

Process	Considerations
Setting up the conversation	*Introduce yourself* – Skip this step if you know the person fairly well. Consider in this part of the process warmth, friendliness, body language, tone of voice. Do you know the person? Do they know you? Have you explained who you are and what your role is? *Confidentiality* – Take the time to explain what you will and won't share and with whom, explain the limits of confidentiality (according to policy) and why this is important. This step makes clear to the service user where the limits are and allows informed choice about what they do and don't share with you; again it supports the person to feel more in control. *Deciding and exploring what the meeting is for* – Use this opportunity to set up a shared understanding of what the conversation is for, focusing on what you are hoping to achieve (assessment, understanding, planning etc.). Seeking to understand things from the service user's point of view, eliciting and understanding their goals and why and what the service user wants will set a framework for your conversation and allow them to be a partner in the process, ensure they are heard and may reduce any potential anxiety about what they (and you) are there for. *Set the timeframe and give an exit option to the person* – Discuss how long you have for the conversation. Say if you may be interrupted. Explain that they can stop at any time if they wish and give explicit permission for them to do so. This helps the person to feel more in control and gives them permission to interrupt and have a break if needed. It also supports safety for you as the person is more likely to say if they are getting frustrated. *'Difficult conversations': giving permission* – You may be about to talk about some sensitive topics; it can be helpful to say that this may be difficult for the service user (and for you) and that they are free to say if they don't want to discuss something or to let you know that they are finding something difficult. It is also helpful to give a rationale as to why you are doing this and how it may help you to work more effectively with the person; allow them more control and again support safety. You may want to give explicit permission for the person to tell you if they are getting frustrated or if you are not making sense to them, to give you a chance to reframe questions. *Check in and proceed* – Check that the person has understood all of the above and that they are happy to proceed.
During the conversation	*Relax, be yourself and listen* – Pay attention to the key skills and concepts outlined earlier in the chapter. Use active listening, summarise and reflect back to the service user what you have heard, think about your body language and tone of voice. Check that you have understood what they are saying and what it means to them.

Towards the end of the conversation	*Summarising, planning and following up* – Tell the person you are going to summarise what you have discussed and invite them to comment on the accuracy of what you have said and if they think your interpretation is accurate. This allows you to check your understanding, shows you have listened, ensures that the person gets a chance to highlight any inaccuracies and helps you to remember and highlight the key points raised. When care planning this allows you to ensure the goals are mutually agreeable and appropriate. Discuss the next steps and when you will next check in. *Check in and close* – Towards the end of the conversation check in with the person, are they okay? Is anything bothering them or is there anything they would like to add or comment on?
After the conversation	Reflect on what was said, how you think the conversation went and what you think it means. Are there any key issues you need to follow up on or can take away in terms of your own learning? How you are feeling about the process – do you need to seek some supervision? Then write up your notes, sharing with others as needed, and begin acting on the plans made or issues brought up in the conversation.

Table 3.1: Steps to consider when setting up recovery conversations

Challenges to recovery-focused nursing care

The development of a recovery-focused, hope-inspiring relationship within mental health services has a number of potential barriers which need to be recognised and overcome in the first instance. For example, nurses often work within a health care system which may be heavily reliant upon clinical outcomes and symptom reduction as measures of success.

The previous experience of the service user within mental health services will impact on the starting point of this relationship, as well as the difficulties they may be currently experiencing within the context of their current mental health problems (Trenoweth and Larter, 2008). The underlying dynamic that the service user is receiving care within a setting which can forcibly detain and treat that person against their will is likely to have a negative impact on the formation of a truly collaborative relationship, regardless of whether that person is currently receiving compulsory treatment or not. The underlying threat to the free will of the service user does not go unnoticed and cannot be ignored by the clinician. If the nurse has an awareness of this power differential but also recognises that this doesn't mean that he/she is in a position to know what is best for that individual, and that there is a need to promote collaboration within the constraints of these dynamics, a partnership remains achievable where mutual respect for the differing positions may exist. Clearly, a nurse cannot act outside of the rule of the law, or outside of his/her 'duty of care' where the goals of the service user may appear to require this. The role of the nurse within these circumstances would be to offer an honest response to these dilemmas within the context of the conversation, but to also facilitate a discussion about how these goals might be achieved over time, by breaking them down into smaller steps and stages which can be addressed as the larger goal is worked towards (Slade, 2009b).

The longer term impact of coercive treatment and care may be arguably positive in a few cases, where the person is unable or unwilling to fully appreciate the negative effect that his or her behaviour may be having on themselves or those around them at the time. In these circumstances there is clearly an argument for professionals to free the service user of their personal responsibility and to take control of the person, in their best interests. The consequences of them not adopting this paternalistic responsibility could lead to potentially catastrophic consequences for that person's future health and wellbeing and for others. The experience of others taking control away and moderating the person's actions by detaining them in hospital or even enforcing medication against their will, where handled in a sensitive and respectful manner, can be the turning point at which a person later accepts that this was necessary at that time. It is, of course, naive to suggest that at the time the service user will be prepared to appreciate that the actions of the service providers, and more specifically in these situations, the nurses, has been in their best interests, and that the foundations of a collaborative relationship can begin in these moments. In these coercive moments, however, a key aspect remains the quality of the open dialogue and the respectful relationship, whereby honesty and attempting to engage the person in a full explanation of the options open to them as well as encouraging them to be as engaged in the decision-making process as is possible at the time are the underpinning principles when supporting recovery.

There are 'knotty' issues that often remain unresolved in recovery-orientated practice. Some are systemic such as embedded electronic systems for recording clinical information that are often not seen as recovery orientated. There may also be discharge targets or other targets to consider. Other factors may include a seeming clash of values or unresolved issues such as the fundamental recovery principle of 'choice', which includes treatment preferences. The question that often hangs silently in the air is that of whose choice is paramount when there is disagreement. It is important to acknowledge that there may be legal limitations on choice, such as statutory constraints (forensic sentences or the Mental Health Act (MHA)) or periods of loss of capacity affecting decisions when someone is very unwell when it is appropriate to take decisions for that person. Recovery nonetheless requires workers to maximise choice regardless of the situation, and within the constraints, and not to hold onto power over a person's choices once they have regained capacity. The importance of offering choice and empowering individuals to make their own decisions, regardless of how small those choices might appear to the health care professional, should not be underestimated. The ability to think about each situation independently with the service user, and to critically reflect on practice, supports the health professional in their endeavours to support recovery and to minimise the potential harm inflicted by **institutionalisation** (Drennan et al., 2014).

Activity 3.4   *Reflection*

Consider an example of a nursing situation from your personal experience where the service user and the nurse have had opposing views on 'what is best'. How was this resolved? What might have been the impact on that relationship?

Resistance to change

Another difficult issue can be resistance to different ways of working by individuals, teams or the organisation, or a clash of cultures between one or more of those, leading to a dysfunctional culture that is destined for internal confusion or conflict. This can seem an untenable situation for workers and a pressure to resist culture change. The use of some of the MHA terminology, for example, in itself underpins the paternalistic imbalance of power within mental health services. The use of the term responsible clinician can be used to illustrate the continuation of the pervading medical model within mental health services, and arguably seeks to reinforce the power imbalance in the system (Cromer-Hayes and Chandley, 2015). The use of the term 'responsible' could serve to discourage a collaborative approach to positive risk taking and to supporting service users in their own choices and personal responsibility. The title **'responsible clinician'** places the burden of liability and accountability for another directly with that person, and is therefore in complete contrast to the concept of recovery within mental health services. However, the title responsible clinician remains the language of the legal principles underpinning these services, as do the principles of duty of care for all those working with people with mental health difficulties. Professionals are viewed by the wider public as being those with the required knowledge, skills and expertise to care for their service user group, and are publicly blamed for the actions of those in their care when tragedies do occur. It is these public expectations and perceptions which can add additional tension for professionals who work closely with individuals in need of new and innovative methods of working for their own personal longer term growth to help overcome their difficulties. The public's apparent need for the reassurance that people with mental health problems are restricted and managed in a paternalistic and controlling manner reinforces their stigmatisation and social exclusion.

Overcoming barriers to recovery

The nurse may be required to listen to uncomfortable narratives about the service user's personal experiences at the hands of the mental health system, and to build the bridges necessary to move forward with the person. Unpleasant previous experiences or lack of personal control over a situation may manifest as anger and frustration on the part of the service user, or even as aggression towards the clinician or the environment. These situations require support from clinical colleagues and a space for all those involved to reflect upon what has led to this behaviour. The response within a recovery-focused approach also requires an acceptance of personal responsibility by the service user. This understanding requires work from both parties and a continued commitment to a collaborative working relationship. All too often the response of staff is to avoid the individual, chastising them for their unacceptable behaviour, and to seek a remorseful apology, thus reinforcing the power imbalance. A more recovery-focused response would be to offer the service user the opportunity to talk about what has led them to these reactions and how they would like to be cared for or approached in future. This approach will be likely to support the service user in dealing with these frustrations in a more constructive way. A plan which is mutually agreed between service user and clinician in relation to what the service user finds frustrating or difficult to manage, how this may manifest itself as emotions rise, at what point and how he or she would like members of the clinical team to intervene, and how this might be communicated between the two parties would facilitate a more harmonious relationship. It lends itself to a 'personal responsibility' acceptance and makes some strides towards ensuring that the joint working is genuinely based on shared understanding and ownership of goals and required interventions. In this way, a service user can actively support the nurse in drawing up a comprehensive assessment of their risk, and drive the risk management agenda which would be most appropriate for them. It requires clinicians to make a real leap of faith into a working philosophy whereby they trust the service user to identify their own current difficulties and to work with them towards a common aim. This won't work if the aim, or goal, is driven by the agenda of the nurse in the first instance. The key to this collaborative relationship is for the nurse to demonstrate a willingness to work towards whatever the service user feels is in their best interests. Once this message has been conveyed and the relationship moves forward as a partnership, the clinician is in a far better position to seek collaboration and equal personal responsibility in working together to support some of the professional requirements around demonstrating duty of care and the need to practise within any required legal framework (Shepherd et al., 2008).

As a consequence of the prevailing pressures on mental health nurses it could be suggested that all too often first interactions with service users are hijacked by bureaucratic targets, and a requirement to document specific clinical information. Those first conversations cannot later be retracted, and to spend that precious, irretrievable and pivotal engagement opportunity entrenched in a fact-finding dialogue to enable the nurse to complete all of the necessary risk assessment and initial care planning requirements of their clinical setting is in contrast to the collaborative requirements of a truly therapeutic relationship. In addition to these 'targets' the ever-present influence of time constraints on the nurse may dictate that the interaction not only has an agenda, but also that this agenda will hijack the overall dialogue, offering little space and opportunity for the service user to lead the conversation for any length of time in order to express their own concerns, questions and identify their personal priorities for care. This initial interaction will undoubtedly dictate the basis for their ongoing relationship, and for the nurse it is essential that the quality of the engagement is not lost in this clinically driven pre-set agenda. The skill of this initial meeting requires the nurse to elicit any required contextual information whilst ensuring that the dialogue remains service user focused and the personal meaning behind their current experiences can be shared and understood within their social context, any personal distress expressed and their future goals both within the service provision and outside of it can be explored. Clearly, this is highly skilled clinical work, which requires competence, commitment to the foundations of a recovery-focused relationship, and confidence on the part of the nurse. In addition to these key elements, the nurse needs to demonstrate a clear enthusiasm for his/her work to the service user, to convey the importance of that person's current situation to him/her, and the confidence that this can, and will, improve if they work together in a common aim (Slade, 2009a).

Activity 3.5   *Reflection*

Consider a time from your own personal experience when you felt that you weren't being listened to, or when your opinion appeared to be insignificant to the person you were talking to. How did this make you feel and behave?

As nurses we must not lose sight that a person may be a service user but they are also a friend, a son or a daughter and will have a number of other roles. The vast majority of their life takes place outside of mental health services. This may seem self-evident but it is easy to forget, particularly in inpatient services, and also to overestimate our own importance in this person's life. They are at the centre of their life and that life is not located in the centre of our services.

Service user comment: The value of power and control over decision-making

Nothing could have prepared me for ending up in a psychiatric hospital at the age of 21. I didn't want to accept the diagnosis of bipolar affective disorder, or what it would mean for my life; yet I was expected to. My prognosis was grim; I wouldn't go back to university and I wouldn't work – my hopes for the future effectively wiped out. Why would anyone willingly accept this? I had a serious mental health problem that would mean I would take medication for the rest of my life; or so I was told.

The solution to my problems apparently lay in medication and lowering my expectations. The cause of all this was a chemical imbalance in my brain – what could I do about that? While the diagnosis gave me some way to start to make sense of what had happened to me, it left me feeling powerless. In the end I took medication out of fear. 'You will become more unwell if you don't take it, and it will take you longer to get better. You will relapse if you stop taking it.' What else was there if I didn't take this?

My 'problem' was my hopes for the future – when I had resurfaced sufficiently from crippling depression to have any – were deemed unrealistic; every last one of them. This was a challenge I faced over the following 12 years when I used nearly every mental health service that was available, spending more than 3 years of my life admitted somewhere.

I have come to believe that what happened to me had its foundation in childhood trauma, but very few people wanted to have that conversation. I suppose it is more comfortable to talk of chemical imbalances,

(continued)

(continued)

symptoms and to tweak this and that, than to sit with my pain, but the latter was what I needed. The opportunity to do this was offered by voluntary sector therapy provision and later self-funded therapy. I saw an NHS clinical psychologist for a year or so, but I wasn't allowed to see her during my longest hospital admission of 10 months and I was discharged whilst in a recovery house facing totally rebuilding my life. Therapy and just talking to others is where I found my healing; it took a long time and I'm still working on it. Thankfully I met people working within CMHTs and local charities who helped in this process and others who had experienced similar things.

The cycle of severe mental illness is a horrendously tedious thing. What I slowly built up around me came crashing down so many times and I had to start again. I had to turn around a defeated, negative mindset, faced with what often seemed like insurmountable hurdles. I had lost so much; I was ashamed of myself and angry at how my life had ended up. I was painfully aware of how my life differed from the acceptable norm. I became my diagnosis and lost my identity. I was isolated and tried to end my life, amidst a regime of medication, ECT and hopelessness.

Then someone told me repeatedly that I wasn't going to metamorphosise into a completely different person overnight; it would take time, lots of time! It was OK not to be doing what everyone else was doing and it was OK to take time to recover. I didn't have to do what everyone else seemed to be doing. I have done in my late thirties what others did in their twenties, but better late than never!

Sexual dysfunction, weight gain, disabling sedation, memory loss (to name but a few); these are all acceptable things in a world where a pill is heralded as the solution (ECT when the pills don't work). 'She lacks motivation, sleeps the day away, smokes and drinks tea – that's it.' 'Eat less', the psychiatrist told me after I ballooned with the help of olanzapine, while refusing to change it despite my repeated pleas. Thankfully some years later a crisis team psychiatrist heard me and prescribed Quetiapine, which wasn't quite so bad.

When planning my leaving the recovery house, my social worker wanted me to move into supported housing. She was a good and caring person, but she could not support me in my desire to live alone. She withdrew her support and left me to fend for myself in applying and being assessed for social housing. I had recently made a near fatal suicide attempt, and her fears around that were likely her motivation. She visited me in my flat afterwards, but I really needed her support before that.

Later I met a locum consultant psychiatrist who blew me away with his collaborative approach when I went to him having realised that my antidepressant caused sexual dysfunction. I expected him to dismiss my concerns, as had happened so many times before, but he apologised for the side effects of psychiatric drugs, and we took turns in discussing what was going on for me. Did I need an antidepressant? What were my options? On agreeing that I would take an antidepressant, which one was preferable to me? Essentially I had a choice between likely increased appetite or sexual dysfunction, but it was my choice at last. Power and control over decision-making only came in recent years. A feeling of being 'done to' prevailed for too long.

My values and beliefs have changed enormously over this time period and they had to in order to come through this. I had to learn to accept what happened, how I behaved and the impact it had on those who cared for me. I had to forgive my parents who could not teach me what they did not know themselves.

I had to forgive myself. The acceptance and compassion I slowly developed for myself was given to me by others who were often paid to support me. Over the last couple of years I have been reducing the medication that I have taken for 18 years. I don't know if I will ever be free from medication; my primary aim is to keep what I have built. I do feel some resentment that in all that time there was never an attempt to reduce or take me off some of the drugs, but apparently you can't 'rock the boat'.

My life has changed beyond the expectations of myself and others. Every milestone was a white knuckle ride, but thankfully key people walked beside me whilst I developed more positive coping mechanisms and pushed through. From someone who was expected to be on the scrap heap, I am now a voluntary sector manager. I have healthy relationships and I have discovered skills I never knew I had. My stubbornness and perseverance was invaluable, but I'm not sure there would have been enough of that had I not found people who held hope for me when I had none. Those who saw a future for me and believed I could achieve the things I dreamed of. They saw abilities in me that I don't know I had, and I am eternally grateful to them for that. They rekindled the flame that a lack of belief in recovery had nearly blown out.

Author's comment: The value of power and control over decision-making

This service user's journey through her mental health problems has been highly variable both in the meanings attributed to her experience but also in the personal control and opinion she was able to employ. In terms of the key recovery values of hope, control (agency) and opportunity, these were not present in the first years of her journey. This bright, vibrant young woman was therefore deprived of the belief that things would improve and indeed flourish, despite her own immense powers of determination to surmount the difficulties. Part of the story represents an entrenched and hopeless belief that things were as they were and would remain so. The latter part of the story has been driven by her and she has found, often against strongly resistant positions, that she is now leading her care plan and it would seem from my external position as friend and colleague that she is using services and therapies to support her life, not the other way round. She has not confined herself to the somewhat limited therapeutic choices of the NHS, as experienced by her. She has additionally chosen other approaches such as counselling, volunteering, education, physical exercise and many more. This is important if recovery is going to discuss choice in person-led care planning as a reality.

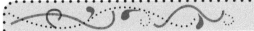 Chapter summary

In this chapter, we have explored ways of delivering recovery-focused care and discussed the difficulties that may arise both for us as professionals and for service users in need of that care. Some people are more resilient than others and we have discussed the ways in which hope, optimism and a sense of retaining some control may be related to a person's recovery.

(continued)

continued . . . . •

We have looked at strategies and approaches for positive engagement with service users including Rogers' person-centred therapy and the counselling technique of motivational interviewing.

We have discussed how we might identify the barriers to developing recovery-focused therapeutic relationships, including resistance to change (on the part of professionals, service users, families and the wider society), and have looked at the importance of communication to support relationship building. Readers have been encouraged to develop their listening skills and look at positive ways of structuring recovery conversations.

Recovery narratives and personal stories from service users have been an important feature of the chapter, helping us to keep their perspective always within view.

Activity: Brief outline answer

Activity 3.3: Reflection (pages 38–9)

You probably noted that the person was attentive in their body language, they were looking at you, they were facing you, they were not distracted, they were not steering the conversation to another topic. They were most likely asking you questions about what you were saying, repeating parts of what you had said and were nodding or shaking their head. Perhaps they were laughing if the story was amusing or expressing empathy to you if this was a difficult situation. You were unlikely to feel you were being judged by the person; if you did feel this you may not have told them the story. In short they were interested in you and wanted to know what you were saying and what it meant to you.

Further reading

ACAS (2014) *Promoting positive mental health at work*. Available at: www.acas.org.uk/media/pdf/1/a/Promoting_positive_mental_health_at_work(SEPT2014).pdf

Slade, M. (2013) *100 ways to support recovery: A guide for mental health professionals* (2nd edn). Available at: www.rethink.org/media/704895/100_ways_to_support_recovery_2nd_edition.pdf

Useful websites

www.time-to-change.org.uk Time to Change.

www.mind.org.uk Mind.

www.sane.org.uk SANE.

www.rcpsych.ac.uk Royal College of Psychiatrists.

Chapter 4
Promoting social inclusion

Nicky Lambert and Sandra Connell

NMC Standards for Pre-registration Nursing Education

Domain 1: Professional values

2.   All nurses must practise in a holistic, non-judgmental, caring and sensitive manner that avoids assumptions, supports social inclusion; recognises and respects individual choice; and acknowledges diversity. Where necessary, they must challenge inequality, discrimination and exclusion from access to care.

2.2.   Mental health nurses must practise in a way that addresses the potential power imbalances between professionals and people experiencing mental health problems, including situations when compulsory measures are used, by helping people exercise their rights, upholding safeguards and ensuring minimal restrictions on their lives. They must have an in depth understanding of mental health legislation and how it relates to care and treatment of people with mental health problems.

Domain 4: Leadership, management and team working

4.   All nurses must be self-aware and recognise how their own values, principles and assumptions may affect their practice. They must maintain their own personal and professional development, learning from experience, through supervision, feedback, reflection and evaluation.

Essential Skills Clusters

Care, compassion and communication

2.   People can trust the newly registered graduate nurse to engage in person-centred care empowering people to make choices about how their needs are met when they are unable to meet them for themselves.

4.   People can trust a newly qualified graduate nurse to engage with them and their family or carers within their cultural environments in an acceptant and anti-discriminatory manner free from harassment and exploitation.

Organisational aspects of care

9.   People can trust the newly registered graduate nurse to treat them as partners and work with them to make a holistic and systematic assessment of their needs; to develop a personalised plan that is based on mutual understanding and respect for their individual situation promoting health and well-being, minimising risk of harm and promoting their safety at all times.

> ## Chapter aims
>
> After reading this chapter you should be able to:
>
> - consider the impact of social exclusion for people with mental health issues;
> - discuss the concept of social inclusion in the context of mental health;
> - understand ways of working dynamically to promote social inclusion in partnership with personal and professional support networks.

Introduction

This chapter begins with a discussion on the meaning of **social inclusion** and **social exclusion**, followed by a consideration of key concepts that may impact your practice. The link between social inclusion and recovery is considered at points throughout, and we will explore how social inclusion can be facilitated.

The context of social exclusion

It may seem contradictory to start this chapter on social *inclusion* by discussing social *exclusion*; however, understanding how social exclusion impacts people can encourage inclusive practice. Thinking about what good practice means in regards to these concepts can challenge our expectations of the boundaries between health and politics and our personal views on individual responsibility – it is not always comfortable, but it is important to think about.

Social exclusion and inclusion are concepts that have been a feature of government policy over the past two decades in the UK. In 1997, the New Labour Government set up the Social Exclusion Unit (SEU), aimed to improve governmental action to reduce social exclusion, not just for those with mental health problems, but for specific groups of people at risk of exclusion. It was designed to address reintegration of marginalised groups, to stop further exclusion and ensure equal service delivery. In 2004, a report by the SEU on mental health and social exclusion highlighted the extent of the issue for people with mental health problems and an action plan was developed to address two key questions: *What needed to be done to assist people with mental health problems entering and retaining work?* And: *How can the same opportunities for access to services and social participation be realised for people with mental health problems?*

It stated the importance of changing public perception, offering early support and choice, sustainable employment, social participation and a collaborative approach between services (Office of the Deputy Prime Minister (ODPM), 2004). Although the Social Exclusion Unit is no longer in existence, we have seen the targeting of social exclusion as a consistent feature of publications including, but not limited to:

- **The Ten Essential Shared Capabilities** (DH, 2004) – Developed as a framework to guide training and curriculum of staff working in mental health services, the capabilities included challenging inequality, working in partnership and respecting diversity.

- **Capabilities for Inclusive Practice** (DH, 2007) – Good practice guidance for staff working in mental health. These were adapted from the Ten Essential Shared Capabilities.

- **Fair Society, Healthy Lives** (Marmot Review, 2010) – Focused on reducing health inequalities and recommended objectives included creating fairer employment and a healthy standard of living for all.

- **No Health Without Mental Health: A cross government mental health outcomes strategy for people of all ages** (DH, 2011) – Aimed at improving the population's mental health and wellbeing, as well as targeting high quality services' accessibility, improving outcomes for those with mental health problems and reducing stigma and discrimination.

- **Closing the Gap: Priorities for essential change in mental health** (DH, 2014) – These actions included tackling inequalities in accessing mental health services, and improving the quality of life for people with mental health problems.

- **The Five Year Forward View for Mental Health** (Mental Health Taskforce, 2016) – Identifies priority actions including creating mentally healthy communities and working with local and national government to increase people's to access services and recognition as equal participants in their communities.

What is social exclusion?

Activity 4.1	*Reflection*

Take a few moments to consider what you think social exclusion means, and note down the words you associate with it.

There is an outline answer at the end of this chapter.

Social exclusion is a complex experience which, like *recovery*, is specific and personal. The Royal College of Psychiatrists (RCP, 2009) noted wider consequences to exclusion; they describe it as a 'blight' on society, and they state people want the opportunity to participate but can be excluded from valuable social roles – that could be anything from voting to home ownership. Often in nursing we look at what an individual can do to change or recover – another way to understand the issues of social exclusion is to think about the ways that society needs to be different to be fair, inclusive and to offer social justice.

In their review of literature on social exclusion, Morgan et al. (2007) found that while there was no universal definition of social exclusion, there are commonalities. The ODPM (2004) describes social exclusion as the experience of multiple, interrelated problems including unemployment, ill health, poverty, poor housing, and lack of skills, illness and stigma. Indeed (Wright and Stickley, 2013) also refer to social exclusion being associated with poverty, unemployment, inequality and disadvantage. More broadly it has been defined as an inability to participate in key areas of public life which stems from external forces rather than personal choice (Berry et al., 2010). This could be people with mental health issues getting meaningful jobs, being seen as electable for public office or being fairly approved for loans or insurance. Levitas et al. (2007) add that relationships and activities across economic, social, cultural and political areas which are available to the majority of society are denied, or lack in availability for those experiencing social exclusion. That could be everything from people with mental health issues being seen as good neighbours or tenants, to being recognised as potential romantic partners or friends.

Most definitions of social exclusion include marginalised people being prevented from participating in multiple areas of life. However, there is no agreement on which dimensions are the most relevant, or if multiple disadvantage is necessary and whether any one of the dimensions is enough to classify someone as socially excluded (Morgan et al., 2007). This returns us to an earlier point that social exclusion is unique to the individual and that we need to consider the personal experience rather than rely on objective markers of social exclusion.

Activity 4.2 — *Critical thinking*

Social exclusion can relate to areas of personal, financial and social life. Make a list under each word on how an individual might be affected.

PERSONAL	FINANCIAL	SOCIETAL

There is an outline answer at the end of this chapter.

The Royal College of Psychiatrists (RCP, 2009) highlighted that:

- *Exclusion is profoundly negative; it affects society as a whole.*

- *People want to participate or at the least, feel that they belong in their societies; exclusion is not a natural state – it is brought about by someone or something.*

- *People who are excluded often suffer from multiple disadvantages, for example social disadvantage, poverty, mental health problems and intellectual disability.*

- *Although there are strong associations between poverty, disadvantage, deprivation, exclusion and mental ill health – these are not fixed states; they can fluctuate and be modified.*

Social inclusion

By now, you should have a clearer understanding of what social exclusion means and the detrimental effect it can have on multiple areas of a person's life. However, it is not enough to see social inclusion as doing the opposite of social exclusion; knowing the approaches and values inherent to practice that promote social inclusion is important, but tailoring these to meet the specific needs of the individuals you work with brings about practice that has integrated and been moulded by both social inclusiveness and recovery. For example Shepherd et al. (2008) highlights the importance of mental health workers using a full range of community resources to support mental health recovery, which furthers the opportunity for people to access, contribute and gain from communities they live in.

As with social exclusion, social inclusion is not an easily definable term. Perhaps a useful place to begin with is with Sayce (2001) who described it as including improved rights of access to society, better opportunities for participation, and the recognition of personal meaning and status.

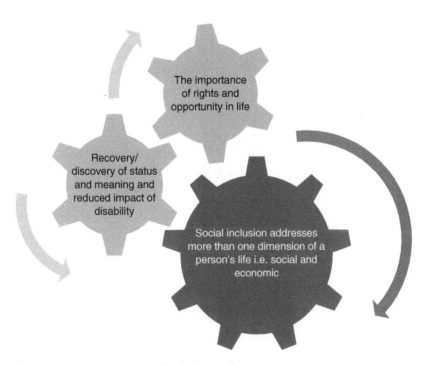

Figure 4.1: The relationship between social inclusion and recovery

Clifton et al. (2013, p159) goes beyond this expectation saying that social inclusion means not only that people are tolerated, but they are safe and welcomed in communities:

> *... is the notion that people experiencing mental health problems are accorded the same rights and opportunities as all fellow citizens. They should be able to participate in every aspect of society without fear of discrimination.*

Working in a socially inclusive way

Working in a socially inclusive way means paying attention to the different areas of a person's life guided by the level of importance they attach to different areas – so we are working together towards the same goals. There are benefits for a number of parties to working in a socially inclusive way (RCP, 2009), including:

- **Service users, carers and professionals:** Better outcomes may be experienced by the individual with the focus on their preferences and needs, as well as development of collaborative relationships.

- **Economic benefits:** The cost of social exclusion is not just to the individual, but to families and wider society. Addressing areas such as improving access to employment means increased financial security for individuals but also potentially increases tax contributions to government revenue, and could decrease spending on care as health improves.

- **Social benefits:** Improved opportunity of access to socially supportive networks may help in terms of the person's mental health, but also their sense of being part of a community.

Shepherd et al. (2014) developed guidance for supporting recovery at the individual level which also included quality indicators such as access to housing and employment, while Roberts and Boardman (2014) in their article focusing on recovery-orientated practice identified the need for 'developing natural supports and promoting community participation'; both of which demonstrate how recovery working encompasses social inclusion.

However, the empirical evidence base to support social inclusion and mental health is minimal which means that the development of meaningful interventions for practice is difficult (Wright and Stickley, 2013). This has led to suggestions that rather than focusing on specific actions, or interventions, best practice is working in a way that reduces health inequalities and promotes individual rights. Berry et al. (2008) also remind us that by targeting stigma and seeking equal and meaningful participation for those we work with, we can promote changes to society, rather than just locating the source of 'difficulty' solely in the individual.

Aslan and Smith (2012) explored a wider, more political perspective on health by considering how social inclusion necessitates 'meaningful occupation and social restoration' (p195). This highlights the importance of not just working with the individual which is a recognised expectation for practitioners, but tackling societal issues which can take us outside of our comfort zone.

Indeed practising in a socially inclusive way is not without its complications and areas of conflict:

- *We are working from the assumption that people want to be included in a society that they have experienced the negative effects of exclusion from (Clifton et al., 2013). This is not always the case although people must always have the option to participate.*

- *To imply that action is only required at the individual and societal level is ignoring the need for action at the level of service provision. Staff may have the values and practical ability to work in a socially inclusive way, but if this is not facilitated by organisational structure or service philosophy, this may lead to conflict for staff in meeting the requirements of their role. As noted previously in this chapter, we have seen that social inclusion has been part of governmental plans and policy for two decades, which implies some wider political response to the need for social inclusive services.*

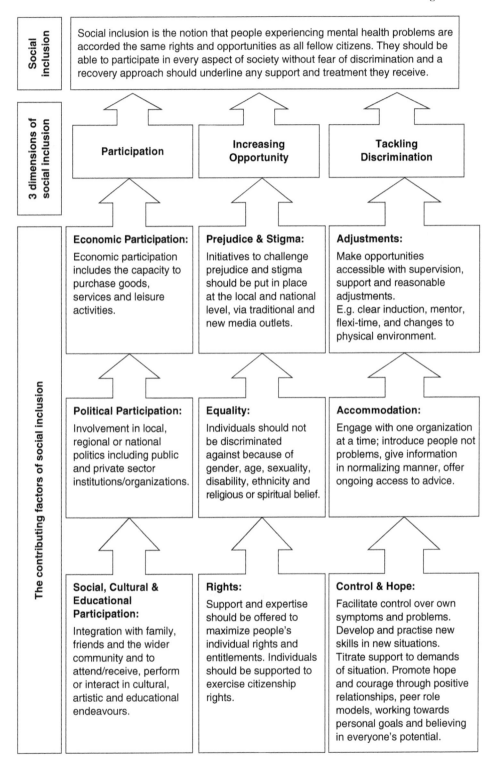

Figure 4.2: Reproduced with permission from Clifton, A., Repper, J., Banks, D. and Remnant, J. (2013) Co-producing social inclusion: The structure/agency conundrum, Journal of Psychiatric and Mental Health Nursing, 20: 519

Figure 4.2 proposes a framework for consideration by health care professionals and nurses when working to increase social inclusion. This allows us to see three key overarching areas of action (participation, increasing opportunity and tackling discrimination).

Social inclusion, society, health and recovery

Promoting inclusion, and paying attention to and advocating for people's rights in society requires an understanding of a person's experience in life, as does facilitating recovery. Working with a person to discover their strengths and what they want from their life facilitates personal recovery, but needs to consider all aspects of the person's life. Roberts and Boardman (2014) note challenges given that the priorities for the individual may not necessarily be the focus of the service. This brings us to look at the concept of recovery and related issues.

Recovery is a concept that can take many forms: for example it may be seen as a remission of medically defined symptoms, personal adjustment to, or mastery of the experience of illness and it can also relate to our ability to connect to society and be productive members of society. It is this connection between society and wellness that makes social inclusion and recovery important to consider in relation to practice.

From a social perspective, the idea that recovery has occurred if someone is a *productive* member of society and contributes to the social structure is an interesting one, because it is functionally based rather than rooted in health. Certainly it is not uncommon to use someone's ability to live independently, hold down a job and have relationships as a measure of their wellbeing (see Chapter 5). It is useful to remember though that what is considered socially desirable changes across societies and throughout time. Ideas of what is *normal* and *not normal* are rarely helpful to us when thinking about how to ethically promote an individual's role in society.

Political ideas also shape this discussion, for example in the current climate of austerity in the UK there is a drive to increase the numbers of people in work. One aspect of this strategy is **cognitive behavioural therapy** (CBT) which is being offered in some job centres. Whilst this seems reasonable where being unemployed has caused individuals anxiety or depression, arguably it contains confusing messages about people who have multiple vulnerabilities due to mental health issues and being out of work. There are differences between the way people impaired by illness are being treated in this instance: people with physical health problems are supported via the health system to get well whilst those with mental health issues are 'helped' to get a job. CBT may be linked for some to continuing to receive benefits, which is at odds with the expectations of most talking therapies, and compelling someone to engage in a therapeutic endeavour is at best counterproductive. Most importantly though not being able to get a job in a recession cannot in itself be seen as a symptom of mental illness; medicalising a social ill in this way arguably locates the issue within the individual rather than in wider society and marginalises and isolates people further. Promoting social inclusion may well be about gaining meaningful employment for one individual, but focusing on meaningful participation in the first instance, and what this is for the person – whether employment, engaging with education or engaging with support networks – is more important.

Patel (2015) describes addressing social injustice as a key public mental health strategy, stating that mental health is 'as much about politics and ideology as medicine and science'. There is an expectation for mental health workers to act as advocates within health structures, but the idea that social action is part of advocacy can cause discomfort for professionals who see the source of their influence and authority to stem from being apolitical.

Health care is shaped by the values and concerns of the society it serves, and the organisation of health provision remains a key concern of the electorate. As trusted professionals with experience of the impact of policy on the health of vulnerable people, practitioners should be civically engaged. Robinson (1997) states that politics are no longer taboo for nurses but that's a long way from staff feeling they are relevant to everyday care.

The NMC *Code* (NMC, 2015) makes it clear that professionals must separate their personal and professional beliefs in order to provide the best standard of care; but there is also an expectation that staff will act as an advocate for others. This potential conflict can leave practitioners unsure how to proceed.

Activity 4.3   *Leadership and decision-making*

The activity below provides you with ways to explore how you exercise your professional judgement in these matters. Below is a list of activities; which box would you put them in?

Where do you stand?

As a professional is it OK to:

1. *Go on a protest march against a hospital or service closure?*
2. *Write to your MP about an issue of poor care?*
3. *Help a mental health service user register to vote?*
4. *Tell that person how you intend to vote?*

Yes, this is ok for a registered mental health professional to do:	No, this is not ok for a registered mental health professional to do:
• _____ • _____ • _____	• _____ • _____ • _____

There are outline answers at the end of this chapter.

Politics and power have always shaped mental health. In many cultures to experience mental health problems is to be stigmatised and can result in rejection or social distance from others in a way that a physical issue would not. Goffman (1963) named this phenomenon **spoiled identity** and suggested that it creates prejudice and discrimination for individuals as well as those close to them: family, friends and professionals (Pescosolido, 2013).This problem is reinforced by findings that groups that already have 'lower' positions in hierarchical social structures experience higher rates of mental health problems (Rosenfield, 2012). This suggests that having mental health issues can cause social exclusion but being socially excluded can heighten mental distress.

Brittan and Maynard (1984) note the tendency of societies to objectify stigmatised people – for example, consider the links the media makes between people with mental health issues and violence. Despite evidence that people with mental health issues are more likely to be victims than perpetrators of violent crime (Appleby et al., 2001), television, films and newspaper stories routinely link mental illness to violence and create a damaging stereotype. Not only does stigma of this kind cause unnecessary suffering and may make people afraid to seek help, it also can manifest as social exclusion by reducing acceptance of people with mental health issues in communities. However this stereotype is increasingly challenged by service user-led groups through health promotion initiatives like Time to Change, and such anti-stigma programmes have been found to be broadly successful (Griffiths et al., 2014).

Another way to challenge oppression is to name it, and to understand how it has historically affected people and how they have responded. Audre Lorde (1984) wrote about the *mythical norm* – the belief that there is an ideal standard, that those who make up the dominant culture, those holding societal power in terms of wealth, culture, gender etc. can set the standards for social acceptability and can decide who falls outside it. As a result people who are marginalised in society by factors like poverty, age or poor health can be *othered* (de Beauvoir, 1949), that is seen as something apart and inferior to that which is considered 'normal'. The ugliness of the idea of suggesting another person is socially unacceptable based on an arbitrary difference, like for example mental ill health, is apparent; however it can be resisted and challenged by self-validation and self-definition (Collins, 1986). These ideas might seem far from everyday practice but they are necessary tools for understanding some of the situations you might encounter and ways you could empower the people you work with to challenge unfairness resulting from stigma.

Case studies

- *You are working with Emma, an 18-year-old woman who self-injures sometimes when she is anxious. She tells you she has been asked to leave her local gym because other members have complained that she has scratches on her arms from self-injury.*
- *Dinesh had a recent inpatient stay and although he is feeling well now, he is worried about reconnecting with his friends as they saw him when he was unwell and he is unsure of how they will respond to him.*

Reflecting on the case studies above, the following issues emerge:

- Emma is being denied access to services based on discrimination related to a protected characteristic. Arguably this stems from negative public attitudes and a lack of understanding towards mental distress – it is important that Emma is aware of her legal rights in this situation and your actions would be guided by her wishes.

- Dinesh may be experiencing internal stigma – where the negativity that comes from society can be internalised resulting in his loss of expected social contact. Unfortunately he might be right that his friends reject him and he may need support to overcome this and develop new networks. However it might be his personal fears that need to be overcome in the first instance. Dinesh will guide this process but it may mean exploring his own understanding of his experience of illness and what that means to his sense of self.

Pettie and Triolo (1999) describe the importance of supporting people who are experiencing mental health issues to construct or reconstruct a positive identity and find their place in a world that for many can become unwelcoming. They suggest that there are two types of meaningful identity: that given to us by society and that we choose for ourselves in order to make sense of our lives.

Activity 4.4 — *What makes you, you?*

What social roles do you hold? *(Hint: are you a sister or brother, neighbour, friend, employee, what groups are you a part of etc.)*	What words would you use to describe yourself to someone who hasn't met you?
How would you manage if these roles or descriptions were compromised or taken away from you?	

There is an outline answer at the end of this chapter.

Smith et al. (2015) use narrative and visual arts to support formerly homeless people with complex needs to build their recovery, socially connect and reclaim their identities. However, the smallest things can make a difference at this point in someone's recovery, how you make time to value the people you are working with: using eye-contact, encouragement, listening, unconditional positive regard and the respect that you show can do much to undo the negative messages that can be received from wider society. The therapeutic relationship is key to helping people to remember that they have an important contribution to make to the lives of others. For example, Barker's (2001) **Tidal Model** places interpersonal relations at the heart of nursing practice. It also notes the potential for iatrogenic harm (harm resulting from treatment such as over-medication and including stigma resulting from diagnosis itself).

There are many frameworks available to help practitioners to structure the work they do to support recovery. For example, Barker, Stevenson and Leamy (2000) developed an empowering interactions framework. They suggest that one way to begin to counteract the damage done to people who have been excluded is to make sure that when *you* work with them you do so in a collaborative and respectful way. It is important to remember that they are an expert by experience and that no one else knows more about their life than they do; you should support their capacity to problem solve and make their own decisions as far as possible.

Activity 4.5   *Critical thinking*

Read the case study below and consider what specific actions you could take to make sure that Casey is heard and is respected.

You are working with Casey, a 25-year-old woman who comes to you angry about a story in a newspaper that describes people with mental health issues in a disrespectful way. Reading the article you can see why she is upset as it is discriminatory and offensive; she asks you what she can do about it. How would you respond?

There is an outline answer at the end of this chapter.

Power

A key part of working in a recovery-orientated way is learning to manage power. You may not feel very powerful at work but there are times in your practice where you have to make decisions in someone's best interests and on their behalf – this must be done with care and in the least restrictive way possible. When people make choices and adapt to the consequences of their decisions, they develop a sense of control and can feel empowered.

Jacobson and Greenley (2001) emphasise the value of having control over oneself and describe it as a healing process, noting its importance in reducing the effects of stress. Deegan (1996) writes from her own experience saying 'mental health professionals must not rob us of the opportunity to fail', but there can be contradictions in mental health with conflicting responsibilities to support people's choices to take risks whilst protecting them and the public. It is important to ensure that we allow for positive risk taking where possible and don't promote overly defensive practice. However there are practice areas where it can be difficult to balance the two opposing demands of advocacy and safeguarding – specific guidance such as *Making Recovery a Reality in Forensic Settings* by Drennan and Wooldridge (2014) can prove invaluable in such situations.

Promoting and valuing networks

An active, independent service user movement is one of the best ways to ensure recovery-focused care; it can offer a range of benefits from challenging professional viewpoints and adding a different perspective to decisions. Service users may teach staff as 'experts by experience' and act as role models for people in recovery; as Deegan (1988) notes, someone who is a peer can offer valuable support and practical understanding.

Friends and family can be central in supporting their loved ones' recovery; unfortunately mental health environments are not always welcoming and whilst there are times where a duty of confidentiality means information cannot be shared, often supporters are left confused and worried when their loved ones are in services.

Carers can be subject to stigma and prejudice based on their family members' mental health issues. That stigma can be external – from others which in turn can affect the availability of a socially supportive network for the service user. However, the experience of stigma can also be internal; as members of the public they may have a layperson's level of understanding of the issues. By making sure that carers have information on mental health issues (Mind Info is an accessible place to start) and how to help support recovery, you are promoting social inclusion. After all, the first and most important social group we belong to are the people who we love; if family and friends are unsure of how to help, they can feel overwhelmed and support networks can break down.

The importance of belonging is evident in Leamy et al.'s (2011) work. They use the acronym CHIME to structure ways of working to encourage socially inclusive recovery, and we have suggested actions based on their framework.

	Need	Ways you could help
C	Connectedness	*Supporting family and friends to maintain contact or develop a support system. Keeping jobs and housing secure during periods of mental ill health.*
H	Hope for the future	*Role-modelling the belief that recovery is possible, focusing on strengths, promoting choice and celebrating small steps forward.*
I	Identity	*Making sure people have access to their belongings: especially their own clothes, music etc. Address spiritual needs.*
M	Meaning in life	*Encourage expressions of identity, creativity and purpose. Make time for people to consider their world view and how they fit in – this can change with the experience of being unwell.*
E	Empowerment	*Make sure people know their rights, ensure they have access to independent advocates and challenge stigma in partnership and as a whole team when it is encountered.*

Adapted from Leamy et al. (2011).

Chapter summary

This chapter has explored the practical and psychological impacts of social exclusion for people with mental health issues. It has addressed some of the ideas or concepts that are important in understanding social inclusion in the context of mental health. It has also suggested ways that you could proactively work to promote social inclusion.

(continued)

continued . . . . .

> This last quote from Slade et al. (2014) describes recovery as the 'goal of reclaiming a mean-ingful life – a process that is based on self-determination and respect for the individual as a citizen of society'. It is a good place to end because it encapsulates the important themes of recovery and social inclusion: valuing the individual and their place in the community.

Activities: Brief outline answers

Activity 4.1: Reflection (page 51)

You may have come up with many different words, some of which may relate to the subjective experience such as loneliness and isolation, and some of which refer to a broader objective meaning of social exclusion such as affected areas – economic, housing or health. As we have seen in the chapter, social exclusion is complex to define, but a key issue that is common across definitions is the lack of participation which is not due to personal choice. In addition, social exclusion refers to a number of interrelated problems that can be mutually re-enforceable such as poverty, homelessness and unemployment. The degree to which a person is affected in the varying areas will be personal and specific.

Activity 4.2: Critical thinking (page 52)

There are many examples you could come up with here, for example:

PERSONAL – relationships with family and friends, widening social circles, dating, group memberships.
FINANCIAL – being able to get loans, open bank accounts, make money or have enough to pay the bills and save.
SOCIETAL – having access to leisure activities, education, employment, and being relied on by others or seen as responsible etc.

Activity 4.3: Leadership and decision-making (page 57)

As a professional is it ok to:

1. *Go on a protest march against a hospital or service closure?* – Yes, you can protest as a citizen, but be wary of organisations attempting to use your professional status to add legitimacy to their cause.

2. *Write to your MP about an issue of poor care?* – Yes, you can contact your MP about any issue but you need to make sure that you have followed your trust/organisational Raising Concerns expectations and you need to stay within your code of conduct regarding confidentiality and best practice in terms of reporting failures of care.

3. *Help a mental health service user register to vote?* – Yes; people often misunderstand the law in this respect. People on a mental health section have the right to vote (unless they were sent to hospital by a criminal court, or transferred from prison). They can register for a postal or proxy vote but must register on the electoral register as living either at their hospital address or at a recent home address.

4. *Tell that person how you intend to vote?* – No, even if this takes place in an informal conversation it could be seen as coercive or exerting undue influence on a person in your care.

In order to explore these issues more, you may like to read the following:

Hannigan, B. and Burnard, P. (2000) Nursing, politics and policy: A response to Clifford. *Nurse Education Today*, 20 (7), 519–23.

Robinson, J. (1997) Power, politics and policy analysis in nursing. In: Perry, A. (ed.) *Nursing: A knowledge base for practice* (2nd edn). London: Arnold, pp249–81.

Ryan, S.F. (2015) *Nurse Practitioners and Political Engagement: Findings from a Nurse Practitioner Advanced Practice Focus Group and National Online Survey.* Available at: http://anp-foundation.org/wp-content/uploads/2015/04/Nurse_Practitioners_and_Political_Engagement_Report.pdf.

Woodward, B., Smart, D. and Benavides-Vaello, S. (2016) Modifiable factors that support political participation by nurses. *Journal of Professional Nursing,* 32 (1), 54–61.

Activity 4.4: What makes you, you? (page 59)

The social roles you might have identified include being a family member, part of friendship groups, a neighbour, friend, employee, choir member, dog walker! How you see yourself and how you might cope with your sense of self being challenged or devalued will be personal – recognising how and why these things are important to you can help you empathise and support others in a similar situation.

Activity 4.5: Critical thinking (page 60)

There's no one right way to respond, but things that might help include acknowledging that Casey's feelings are valid. You can also support her to take action; she is not powerless – we all shape the society we live in. Mind offers guidance to complain about inappropriate coverage of mental health: www.mind.org.uk/news-campaigns/minds-media-office/complain-to-the-media/. For complaints about newspaper articles you can contact the editor. If they don't get back to you in a timely manner or if their response is poor, you can complain to the Independent Press Standards Organisation (IPSO). You could support Casey to do this or support her to enlist others to send a joint complaint with other people. Ongoing, if Casey wants to be more involved in service user activism you can help her access local and national service user groups where she can join with others to help change things for the better.

Useful websites

www.mind.org.uk/information-support/ MIND (information and support).

meam.org.uk/ Making Every Adult Matter (MEAM) – a coalition of charities formed to improve policy and services for people facing multiple needs, especially useful for information on people who are experiencing multiple exclusions.

www.recoverydevon.co.uk/ Developing Recovery Enhancing Environments Measure (DREEM) – an outcome measure and research tool to see how 'recovery-orientated' a service is.

www.tidal-model.com/ Tidal Model resources to promote recovery.

Chapter 5
Strengths and mental wellness

Steve Trenoweth and Wasiim Allymamod

NMC Standards for Pre-registration Nursing Education

Domain 1: Professional values

2.   All nurses must practise in a holistic, non-judgmental, caring and sensitive manner that avoids assumptions, supports social inclusion; recognises and respects individual choice; and acknowledges diversity. Where necessary, they must challenge inequality, discrimination and exclusion from access to care.

3.1. Mental health nurses must promote mental health and wellbeing, while challenging the inequalities and discrimination that may arise from, or contribute to, mental health problems.

Domain 2: Communication and interpersonal skills

Field standard for competence

Mental health nurses must practise in a way that focuses on the therapeutic use of self. They must draw on a range of methods of engaging with people of all ages experiencing mental health problems, and those important to them, to develop and maintain therapeutic relationships. They must work alongside people, using a range of interpersonal approaches and skills to help them explore and make sense of their experiences in a way that promotes recovery.

Domain 3: Nursing practice and decision-making

3.   All nurses must carry out comprehensive, systematic nursing assessments that take account of relevant physical, social, cultural, psychological, spiritual, genetic and environmental factors, in partnership with service users and others through interaction, observation and measurement.

4.   All nurses must ascertain and respond to the physical, social and psychological needs of people, groups and communities. They must then plan, deliver and evaluate safe, competent, person-centred care in partnership with them, paying special attention to changing health needs during different life stages, including progressive illness and death, loss and bereavement.

Domain 4: Leadership, management and team working

5.1. Mental health nurses must use their personal qualities, experiences and interpersonal skills to develop and maintain therapeutic, recovery-focused relationships with people and therapeutic groups. They must be aware of their own mental health, and know when to share aspects of their own life to inspire hope while maintaining professional boundaries.

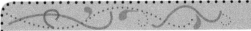

Essential Skills Clusters

Care, compassion and communication

2. People can trust the newly registered graduate nurse to engage in person centred care empowering people to make choices about how their needs are met when they are unable to meet them for themselves.

6. People can trust the newly registered graduate nurse to engage therapeutically and actively listen to their needs and concerns, responding using skills that are helpful, providing information that is clear, accurate, meaningful and free from jargon.

Organisational aspects of care

9. People can trust the newly registered graduate nurse to treat them as partners and work with them to make a holistic and systematic assessment of their needs; to develop a personalised plan that is based on mutual understanding and respect for their individual situation promoting health and well-being, minimising risk of harm and promoting their safety at all times.

Entry to the register

12. In partnership with the person, their carers and their families, makes a holistic, person centred and systematic assessment of physical, emotional, psychological, social, cultural and spiritual needs, including risk, and together, develops a comprehensive personalised plan of nursing care.

Chapter aims

After reading this chapter you should be able to:

* identify factors that support and promote our mental health and protect us from psychological harm;
* describe factors that are related to our mental wellbeing and happiness;
* consider what helps us to flourish and gives a sense of satisfaction, meaning and purpose to our lives.

Introduction

Traditional approaches to mental health care tend to focus on that which is troubling the individual, or, to put this another way, the difficulties and challenges that a person may be facing and what may be going wrong for the person in their life. However, a central idea in the recovery approach is that there needs to be an appreciation of the balance between troubling events and experiences, and how our skills, abilities and assets help us to cope with and manage our current difficulties. In this chapter, we examine this important aspect of the recovery approach and discuss those factors that support and promote our mental health and protect us from psychological harm. We also consider factors that are related to our mental wellbeing and happiness and help us to flourish and give a sense of satisfaction, meaning and purpose to our lives.

Service user comment: What is helpful?

My personal journey started when I was 24 years old, when I was diagnosed with paranoid schizophrenia. I am now 39 years old and an inpatient in a secure hospital where I have been since 2010. I am currently on the discharge pathway and should be returning to life in the community soon. Being in a psychiatric hospital was scary at first, being locked up with other people who are unwell and strangers to me was a difficult experience. I am now on the road to recovery and the things that have helped me get there are: volunteering for charitable organisations, working in the hospital in roles made available to patients to improve skills and confidence, and I am currently studying a horticultural course at the moment in the community. I hope that the medication I am on will keep me stable for the rest of my life as I don't want to return to hospital again after this last 5-and-a-half year stay.

Strengths

Our *strengths* are the resources of ourselves and/or our environment that can *protect* us in times of adversity. Some people have more resources than others. The **Stress Vulnerability Model** (Zubin and Spring, 1977) reminds us of the factors which impact on our ability to cope at times of adversity. In this model, *external stressors* (often caused by significant life events such as deaths, divorce, financial problems and so on) may impact detrimentally on our mental health and wellbeing and challenge our ability to cope. For Zubin and Spring (1977), our response to such stress seems related to our inherited genetic background and to our previous life experiences (such as exposure to parenting styles, trauma, abuse, poor or unhelpful coping mechanisms and so on). Such factors may *predispose* us to mental distress. In particularly vulnerable people, such as those who have ongoing mental health needs, failure to cope with such stresses may place their mental health under strain and increase the likelihood of further mental ill-health or relapse. Conversely, factors such as our coping abilities, helpful beliefs, positive relationships and social networks, personal strengths and talents can reduce our vulnerability to distress at times of crisis and protect us from psychological harm.

Activity 5.1 — *Reflection*

List your skills, abilities and talents. What do you think you are best at? How does this contribute to your happiness and satisfaction with life?

Now, take some time to consider what your vulnerabilities to stress might be. Consider your genetic/family background and life experiences.

The VIA Survey (or VIA Inventory of Strengths) is an assessment instrument that is available free of charge at **www.viacharacter.org**, which measures the 24 character strengths in the individual (Figure 5.1).

Appreciation of beauty and excellence [awe, wonder, elevation]: Noticing and appreciating beauty, excellence, and/or skilled performance in all domains of life, from nature to art to mathematics to science to everyday experience.

Bravery [valour]: Not shrinking from threat, challenge, difficulty, or pain; speaking up for what is right even if there is opposition; acting on convictions even if unpopular; includes physical bravery but is not limited to it.

Citizenship [social responsibility, loyalty, teamwork]: Working well as a member of a group or team; being loyal to the group; doing one's share.

Creativity [originality, ingenuity]: Thinking of novel and productive ways to do things; includes artistic achievement but is not limited to it.

Curiosity [interest, novelty-seeking, openness to experience]: Taking an interest in all of ongoing experience; finding all subjects and topics fascinating; exploring and discovering.

Fairness: Treating all people the same according to notions of fairness and justice; *not* letting personal feelings bias decisions about others; giving everyone a fair chance.

Forgiveness and mercy: Forgiving those who have done wrong; giving people a second chance; *not* being vengeful.

Gratitude: Being aware of and thankful for the good things that happen; taking time to express thanks.

Hope [optimism, future-mindedness, future orientation]: Expecting the best in the future and working to achieve it; believing that a good future is something that can be brought about.

Humour [playfulness]: Liking to laugh and tease; bringing smiles to other people; seeing the light side; making (not necessarily telling) jokes.

Integrity [authenticity, honesty]: Speaking the truth but more broadly presenting oneself in a genuine way; being without pretense; taking responsibility for one's feelings and actions.

Judgement [open-mindedness, critical thinking]: Thinking things through and examining them from all sides; *not* jumping to conclusions; being able to change one's mind in light of evidence; weighing all evidence fairly.

Kindness [generosity, nurturance, care, compassion, altruistic love, 'niceness']: Doing favours and good deeds for others; helping them; taking care of them.

Leadership: Encouraging a group of which one is a member to get things done and at the same time maintaining good relations within the group; organising group activities and seeing that they happen.

(continued)

Figure 5.1 (continued)

Love: Valuing close relations with others, in particular those in which sharing and caring are reciprocated; being close to people.

Love of learning: Mastering new skills, topics, and bodies of knowledge, whether on one's own or formally; obviously related to the strength of curiosity but goes beyond it to describe the tendency to add *systematically* to what one knows.

Modesty and humility: Letting one's accomplishments speak for themselves; *not* seeking the spotlight; *not* regarding oneself as more special than one is.

Persistence [perseverance, industriousness]: Finishing what one starts; persisting in a course of action in spite of obstacles; 'getting it out the door'; taking pleasure in completing tasks.

Perspective [wisdom]: Being able to provide wise counsel to others; having ways of looking at the world that make sense to oneself and to other people.

Prudence: Being careful about one's choices; *not* taking undue risks; *not* saying or doing things that might later be regretted.

Self-regulation [self-control]: Regulating what one feels and does; being disciplined; controlling one's appetites and emotions.

Social intelligence [emotional intelligence, personal intelligence]: Being aware of the motives and feelings of other people and oneself; knowing what to do to fit in to different social situations; knowing what makes other people tick.

Spirituality [religiousness, faith, purpose]: Having coherent beliefs about the higher purpose and meaning of the universe; knowing where one fits within the larger scheme; having beliefs about the meaning of life that shape conduct and provide comfort.

Zest [vitality, enthusiasm, vigor, energy]: Approaching life with excitement and energy; *not* doing things halfway or halfheartedly; living life as an adventure; feeling alive and activated.

Activity 5.2   *Reflection*

How many of the strengths outlined in the VIA Survey do you feel you have? How many would you like to develop?

Now, consider how *hope, zest for life, gratitude, love* and *curiosity* might contribute to your mental wellbeing.

The VIA Classification of Strengths can be helpful for people to understand their characters better and subsequently to take advantage of their positive personal qualities in enhancing their everyday lives (Snyder et al., 2011). However, not all strengths may equally support our mental wellbeing. Of all the many strengths identified in Figure 5.1, it seems that *hope, zest for life, gratitude, love* and *curiosity* are the ones which are most substantially related to satisfaction with one's life (Park et al., 2004).

Mental wellbeing

Activity 5.3	*Critical thinking*

Consider the following questions:

- What keeps you mentally well?
- What contributes to mental health and wellbeing?

In 2010, the prime minister launched the National Well-being Programme. The aim was to measure how our lives are improving. This was not just about standards of living, but our overall quality of life. Since then the Office for National Statistics (ONS) has collated Personal Well-being findings from the Annual Population Survey.

Visit the ONS site for National Well-being (available at: **www.ons.gov.uk/peoplepopulationand community/wellbeing/bulletins/measuringnationalwellbeing/2015-09-23**). Now, consider:

- How is data on personal wellbeing collected?
- How personal wellbeing varies across the country?
- What changes there have been to life satisfaction and happiness?

The survey is clear not to relate happiness with national wealth. Why might this be do you think?

What exactly is **mental wellbeing**? Mental wellbeing is a complex concept but it is generally considered that our mental wellbeing comprises mental health, happiness, hope and optimism and life satisfaction, positive psychological functioning, resilience to adversity, autonomy and a sense of control over one's life, self-awareness and acceptance, and supportive and interpersonal relationships. Moreover, mental wellbeing is a personal experience – it is subjective in that it is something that we feel about ourselves.

For the World Health Organization (WHO), health is 'not merely the absence of disease or infirmity' (WHO, 1946). It further defines mental health as:

> *a state of well-being in which the individual realises his or her own abilities, can cope with the normal stresses of life, can work productively and fruitfully, and is able to make a contribution to his or her community.*
> (WHO, 2007b)

The mental health strategy for England (*No Health Without Mental Health*) describes mental wellbeing as:

> *A positive state of mind and body, feeling safe and able to cope, with a sense of connection with people, communities and the wider environment.*
> (DH, 2011, p90)

These definitions suggest that our mental health and wellbeing is a holistic and personal experience. That is, if we have a positive sense of our own mental wellbeing we may be satisfied with our life overall and we are also likely to have a positive sense of our own physical health. Mental wellbeing also reflects feelings of security and our ability to function, cope within, and make a contribution to society, recognising the social nature of our functioning as human beings.

Despite the challenges of defining mental wellbeing, there have been a number of attempts to capture and measure individuals' perceptions of their own mental wellness. Most recently, the Warwick-Edinburgh Mental Well-Being Scale (WEMWBS) (available at **www.healthscotland. com/documents/1467.aspx**) (Stewart-Brown and Janmohamed, 2008) has been developed with the aim of measuring mental wellbeing among adults over the age of 16 years. This is a 14-item self-report scale capturing perceptions of subjective mental wellbeing and positive mental health during the previous fortnight. Responses are scored on a 1 to 5 Likert scale (where 1 is 'none of the time' to 5 'all of the time'). Scores are summed and the range is 14 to the maximum 70. Higher scores are associated with greater subjective feelings of mental wellbeing.

Activity 5.4   *Evidence-based practice*

Take the Warwick-Edinburgh Mental Well-Being Scale. (Available at: **www.healthscotland. com/documents/1467.aspx**. NB: to view, click 'Read Only'.)

Consider your score. What does this suggest about your own mental wellbeing? Do you agree? What could be done to increase your score, that is, to increase your sense of personal wellness?

Control and autonomy

If we feel that we have positive mental wellbeing we may have a sense of our own personal autonomy in that we feel we have control of and manage our lives and have a sense of being able to rely on ourselves to cope in times of trouble. We may feel we have the competence and relevant skills and abilities and resources to cope with and bounce back after adversity (Ryff, 1989; Ryff and Keyes, 1995). This is known as **resilience** (see below). We may also feel that we can overcome or influence others or our environment, such as by being assertive (Westbrook and Viney, 1980). This is **self-efficacy**, which may be seen as:

beliefs in one's capabilities to mobilise the motivation, cognitive resources, and courses of action needed to meet given situational demands.
(Wood and Bandura, 1989, p408)

However, people who lack a sense of positive mental wellbeing may have feelings of helplessness or consider that they are a victim of circumstance. They may feel at the mercy of external forces (Westbrook and Viney, 1980) and have little hope of being able to reach their goals.

The experience of being in control of our own lives is one which most adults enjoy and take for granted. The ability to take available opportunities and to enjoy a family life or to have a 'working life' which contributes to wider society; to be part of a local community and to have access to services which contribute to a person's sense of security and wellbeing, are all principles which most people hold dear.

The experience of mental ill-health can have a profound effect on all of these aspects of our lives, even to the point of no longer feeling that we have any sense of control over our own life decisions and that our opinion is not only ignored, but worse it is never sought in the first instance (Repper and Perkins, 2003). All experiences change us and reframe our world and the 'illness' experience is just the same. Conversely, the practice of discussing recovery, sharing the knowledge that it is personally defined, acknowledging that people take varying routes and lengths of times and the journey contains setbacks and difficulties but that it is to be expected and supported, is therapeutic and inspiring. Many people will not know this and you may unlock the first empowering door in their recovery.

Personal, meaningful goals

We may also have clear, personal plans and meaningful goals for our life which we feel we can achieve if we try hard enough (Viney, 1986). We may be able to describe a sense of direction, purpose and meaning in our lives.

There may also be an acceptance of ourselves and our life and our personal experiences, along with the highs and lows of life's events and our abilities as well as limitations (Ryff, 1989; Ryff and Keyes, 1995).

Activity 5.5   *Reflection*

Take some time to reflect upon the following points:

- How in control of your life do you feel? How might this undermine or promote your mental health?
- What are your goals for your life? Do you feel able to achieve them?
- How might you feel if you had no aim or purpose in your life? Or if you were unable to achieve those personal goals that you have set for yourself?

Service user comment: Motivation and goals

All of the interactions that [mental health service users] have with professionals should be geared towards aiding their recovery as they have great needs and need positive role models who will not only help them but will act as guides. I myself have therapeutic relationships with a number of people in the

(continued)

(continued)

hospital where I am a patient. For example, my psychologist who I see once a week, is very supportive of me. He always seems to understand me and has good insight into the type of person that I am and what motivates me. I also have an occupational therapist who is very efficient in getting me involved with work and study placements in the community and I have a good relationship with my named nurse too. She always takes the time out to talk to me every week prior to ward round to ask me how I feel about things that have gone on during the week and what I hope will happen in the coming week. They are all very supportive of me and this really helps me a lot.

Positive interpersonal relationships

As suggested by the above definitions, our personal sense of mental wellbeing is also likely to be associated with our positive interpersonal relationships. For many people, positive interpersonal relationships are assets that *protect* them from psychological harm and distress, *promote* their mental wellbeing and satisfaction with life and *support* resilience at times of adversity.

This is likely to involve our ability to establish and maintain positive, warm, close, supportive and trusting interpersonal relationships. For Ryff (1989) and Ryff and Keyes (1995), this also includes an ability to compromise, a sense of empathy and compassion for others, and an understanding of the ebb and flow of human relationships.

Danzinger (1976) identified a classification of positive relationships based on:

*   'Solidarity' (a sense of belonging and interpersonal integration, social acceptance within a community and a common commitment between people and sharing resources).

*   'Intimacy' (people relating to one another as sources of personal satisfaction, including kindness, altruism, love, empathy, attachment).

*   'Influence' (recognising the relevance of social status and standing within a community or group).

Case study

Christine is in her late 60s and has recently been widowed. One of her adult children has emigrated to Australia and has a young family there. The other lives in London, over 100 miles away, and works very long hours in a high-pressure city job. For the last two years of her husband's life, Christine was his carer and this meant she gave up her part-time job and her social activities such as the art club and book group. Now she feels very isolated and has become depressed.

Marta, her community mental health nurse, realises that Christine's sense of isolation is a major problem. She decides to make an effort to try and talk to Christine about what might interest her. She asks about the work she did and the activities she enjoyed but it is a struggle to get much response. Then, on one visit, she asks about a painting hanging on Christine's living room wall. Christine admits that she painted it herself and used to enjoy her art, but she has lost the knack now, and has lost touch with her friends from the group.

Over the next few weeks, Marta asks more about the art group and the people Christine knew. She encourages Christine to begin to make contact again with some of them, and soon they are able to make rejoining the art group a goal to be worked towards.

Personal growth

Mental wellbeing facilitates our personal growth and supports a personally satisfying life, which is purposeful and meaningful, and capable of reaching its full potential (Ryff and Keyes, 1995; Stewart-Brown and Janmohamed, 2008; Jenkins et al., 2008).

There may be a sense of ongoing development as a person (including being open to new experiences and self-improvement). A person may feel that their *talents, knowledge* and *skills* provide *opportunities* for them to meet their *aspirations* or pursue their personal *interests*.

For Csikszentmihalyi (1975), happiness 'flows' from a positive psychological state where our personal skills are optimally and appropriately challenged and tested by tasks in our daily lives. We become so involved and immersed in a task, which tests us, that we lose all sense of time. This allows us to learn, develop and grow as individuals and develop a personal sense of satisfaction in accomplishment.

Happiness

Positive mental wellbeing is often associated with happy, enjoyable experiences (Westbrook, 1976; Viney and Henry, 2002). However, *happiness* is another complex concept and raises a number of important questions. What exactly *is* happiness? Do we all experience happiness in the same way? Do we all use the same criteria in determining our happiness? Does happiness vary between individuals and cultures? Can we ever be truly and permanently happy?

What is clear is that happiness is a personal and subjective experience. Some studies have also revealed that people seem to describe themselves as generally moderately happy. For example, using the 4-item Subjective Happiness Scale (Lyubomirsky and Lepper, 1999) with a possible range of 1.0 to 7.0, the average score for adult American participants is 4.8 (Seligman, 2002), that is, slightly above the average score of 4.0.

There is a debate between those who see happiness as being related to our personality (these are known as *set points* which are seen as relatively stable personal predispositions for happiness) or that our happiness is reflected by our experiences (which may be less stable depending on circumstance) (Snyder et al., 2011).

For Seligman (2002), however, true happiness is an authentic and enduring experience. This is to be compared with the pursuit of hedonistic experiences, characterised by brief pleasures:

> *Momentary happiness can easily be increased by any number of uplifts, such as chocolate, a comedy film, a back rub, flowers or a new blouse.*
> (Seligman 2002, p45)

The type of happiness Seligman (2002) has in mind is one that is genuine and authentic, but also complex, as suggested by his formula:

$$H = S + C + V$$

Here, H is enduring *happiness*; S is the *set range* or the level to which we eventually return after good or bad news; C are the *circumstances* which we find ourselves in which can influence; and V are those *voluntary factors* which we can control.

Seligman (2002) reviewed research over 35 years and identified external circumstances (the C variable in his happiness equation) that can affect our level of subjective happiness. People who live in a wealth democracy (as opposed to an impoverished dictatorship) tend to be happier, as do people who are married; have avoided negative experiences or negative emotions; and those who belong to a religion. Money, health, level of education and race do not appear to have any effect. It appears that it is our subjective attitude towards such circumstances (for example, if we feel personally impoverished or are dissatisfied with our level of health or ability or the things we feel we *should* have) rather than objective criteria (such as how much money we have in the bank, fitness level and so on) which matters most (Seligman, 2002).

Finally, Seligman (2002) considers the influence of those factors which are under our voluntary control (the V variable in his happiness equation) which can influence happiness. Here, Seligman identifies variables relating to our satisfaction with the past (see 'Satisfaction with life' below), present and future (see 'Hope' below). With regards to satisfaction with the present, Seligman (2002) distinguishes between *pleasures* ('delights that have clear sensory or strong emotional components … ecstasy, thrills, orgasm, delight, mirth, exuberance, and comfort' (p102)) and *gratifications* (personally satisfying activities which engage and absorb us, when we are in touch with our strengths).

Satisfaction with life

The Satisfaction With Life Scale (SWLS) (Diener et al., 1985) is a 5-item self-report scale, which respondents rate on a 7 point scale (1 = Strongly disagree; 2 = Disagree; 3 = Slightly disagree; 4 = Neither agree or disagree; 5 = Slightly agree; 6 = Agree; 7 = Strongly agree). The items are listed in Figure 5.2.

Scores range from 5 to 35, with higher scores revealing higher levels of reported satisfaction with life. For those who score the highest range (in the 30–35 range), life is perceived as enjoyable and domains of life (such as work, family and personal development) are going well. Those with high scores may feel that their life is mostly good and may be motivated to improve less

Items:

1. In most ways my life is close to my ideal.
2. The conditions of my life are excellent.
3. I am satisfied with life.
4. So far I have gotten the important things I want in life.
5. If I could live my life over, I would change almost nothing.

Scoring:

30–35 Very high score; Highly satisfied
25–29 High score
20–24 Average score
15–19 Slightly below average in life satisfaction
10–14 Dissatisfied
 5–9 Extremely dissatisfied

Figure 5.2: The Satisfaction With Life Scale (© Ed Diener, Robert A. Emmons, Randy J. Larsen and Sharon Griffin as noted in the 1985 article in the Journal of Personality Assessment)

successful areas of their lives. For people whose scores are average (that is, average within economically developed countries, where most of the population live), life is generally good and there is an air of satisfaction, but there is also room for improvement. Those who feel less satisfied with their lives (in the 15–19 range), there are some small but nonetheless significant areas of life which are a source of dissatisfaction – this may be due to some recent changes which bring temporary dissatisfaction and may improve but for some people such levels of dissatisfaction may lead to personal reflection and some changes to one's life. Amongst people who express dissatisfaction or extreme dissatisfaction with their lives, life has become challenging. There may be significant problems at home or at work, or there may be significant life events such as bereavements, divorce or redundancy. Persistently low life satisfaction may indicate a chronic condition where the person may need support to make positive changes to their life. It might be, for example, that the individual finds it difficult to let go of an unhappy past or is unable to forgive perceived past wrongs (Seligman, 2002).

Activity 5.6   *Evidence-based practice*

Take the *Satisfaction With Life Scale* (© Ed Diener, Robert A. Emmons, Randy J. Larsen and Sharon Griffin as noted in the 1985 article in the *Journal of Personality Assessment*) (available at: **http://internal.psychology.illinois.edu/~ediener/SWLS.html**).

How satisfied are you with your life? How could you improve this if you would like to?

For Diener et al. (1985), one's general satisfaction with life reflects an individual's personal evaluation of those aspects of his or her own life that are seen as important and 'not upon some criterion which is judged to be important by the researcher' (Diener et al., 1985, p71). To this end, the SWLS should be seen as a general starting point for further discussions on sources of satisfaction and dissatisfaction in their lives.

Hope

Hope is an important concept in recovery approaches to mental health care (Kylmä et al., 2006; Cutcliffe and Koehn, 2007) and supports the person's abilities to change and improve their life. Furthermore, hope may also enhance our sense of self-compassion, skills in personal relationships and life satisfaction (Umphrey and Sherblom, 2014).

For Snyder et al. (2011, p185), hope is 'goal-directed thinking in which the person utilises pathways thinking (the perceived capacity to find routes to desired goals) and agency thinking (the requisite motivations to use those routes)'. So, if we are hopeful we have knowledge of our own personally valued goals, which we are motivated to strive for, and a sense of our own ability to positively and persistently work towards those goals. It also follows that hopeful people are likely to have a sense that if one particular route to their goal is blocked or unfruitful, then they will be able to find other pathways. Furthermore, they are likely to have a zest and an optimism that their efforts to goal-attainment will be worthwhile.

Service user comment: Hope and encouragement

Mental health service users who have been discharged from hospital need the support and encouragement from an outreach team in the community to make sure that the service user is progressing in their recovery and being assisted to set goals that are meaningful for the individual. Without this input life in the community can seem daunting and overwhelming and this can have a negative impact on the service user's progression. This support for me has made me feel that I am not alone and that my team understands me and has given me hope for my future and also the motivation to change my life and how I look at my illness. I no longer see it as a hindrance and now see that it makes me who I am. I hope the new generations of mental health nurses remember why they went into the field and that they are able to provide the best support from a caring perspective.

People who engage with mental health services may have lost much hope and some may even have no hope that they can go on to live meaningful, fulfilling lives. One of the core parts of the nurse's role is to hold onto this hope, develop hope with the service user and demonstrate our own hope and belief in them through our care, compassion and dedication; always believing that the service user is doing the best that they can and holding onto hope that they can build a meaningful and fulfilling future. Pat Deegan (1996) summarised her view of hope at an Australian conference:

It is a spirit of hope. Both individually and collectively we have refused to succumb to the images of despair that so often are associated with mental illness … We are refusing to reduce human beings to illnesses. We recognize that within each one of us there is a person and that, as people, we share a common humanity … We share in the certainty that people labelled with mental illness are first and above all, human beings. Our lives are precious and are of infinite value … we will be learning that those of us with psychiatric disabilities can become experts in our own self-care, can regain control over our lives, and can be responsible for our own individual journey of recovery.

Resilience

Resilience is the 'ability to bounce back or positively adapt in the face of significant adversity or risk' (Snyder et al., 2011, p114). Of course, the issue here is to consider what people are actually 'bouncing back' from? Within recovery approaches, we must assume that this is what the individual personally defines as the normal range of functioning rather than what external agencies consider as being the level a person should be functioning at (Snyder et al., 2011).

For Friedli (2009), there are three broad dimensions that support resilience and help to confer protection at times of adversity:

- **Environmental resources**: features of the natural and built environment that support communal capacity for resilience (not discussed in this book).

- **Social resources**: social networks and family life that enhance resilience amongst people and communities (see 'Positive interpersonal relationships' above).

- **Personal emotional and cognitive resources** that support and contribute to developing resilience amongst individuals, such as good mental health (factors which undermine personal resilience include mental distress, low levels of mental wellbeing and neglect of self and others and a range of unhelpful coping mechanisms and self-harming behaviours, including self-sedation and, e.g., self-medication through alcohol and drugs, high fat and sugar consumption).

Problems with strengths and mental wellbeing

There are, of course, many issues to consider when we look at our own strengths and wellbeing. Sometimes it can be easier for us all to recall the qualities, skills, abilities and talents that we don't have than those we do! This can be even more trying for people who are currently experiencing mental distress. Additionally, there may be gender and cultural influences that discourage discussions of such matters.

Discussions about our strengths can lead to important self-discovery that allows us to reflect and positively appraise our skills and talents. The **Johari window** suggests that there are some elements of our self to which we are blind (that is, not known to us, but known to others), hidden (that is, known to us, but not known to others) and unknown (that is, not known to us or others). The process of mental health assessment can, therefore, be potentially revelatory as the individual may become aware of those aspects of self which have been previously blind or unknown to them. Another important element of an assessment of strengths is the potential problem of capturing variables that are subjective. Self-report can be biased and is subject to errors such as imperfect recall of previous and state-dependent memory, the tendency to recall events and experiences better when one is in the same state as when the memories were formed. That is, happy events are best recalled when we are happy, and sad events are easier to bring to mind when we are sad.

It is generally considered that aspects of our personality are relatively stable and enduring over our adult lives in that we return to a 'set-point' following positive and negative experiences. Of course, this does not mean that we cannot develop new strengths and talents or hone existing ones by acquiring new skills and knowledge. However, our strengths may be compromised at different points in our lives by our life experiences and the situations, conditions and contexts in which we find ourselves, and at such times our personal resilience and our ability to cope with life's problems may be compromised (Snyder et al., 2011).

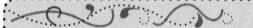

Chapter summary

Traditional approaches to mental health care tend to focus on that which is troubling the individual. However, the recovery approach appreciates the balance between troubling events and experiences, and how our skills, abilities and assets help us to cope with and manage our current challenges. In this chapter we have discussed those factors that assist in protecting us from psychological harm and in promoting our mental health. We also discussed factors that relate to our mental wellbeing, satisfaction and happiness and help us to give a sense of meaning and purpose to our lives. We discussed the concept of mental wellbeing along with strengths, abilities and talents and specific issues of hope, resilience and positive relationships.

Further reading

Seligman, M. (2002) *Authentic happiness.* London: Nicholas Brearley Publishing.

Useful websites

http://ppc.sas.upenn.edu Positive Psychology Center.

www.mind.org.uk/information-support/tips-for-everyday-living/wellbeing/#.V2lLijd5j6Y MIND: How to Improve and Maintain Your Mental Wellbeing.

www.fph.org.uk/concepts_of_mental_and_social_wellbeing Faculty of Public Health.

Chapter 6
Promoting recovery throughout our lives

Rachel Perkins and Phil Morgan

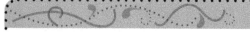

Essential Skills Clusters

Care, compassion and communication

2. People can trust the newly registered graduate nurse to engage in person centred care empowering people to make choices about how their needs are met when they are unable to meet them for themselves.

Organisational aspects of care

9. People can trust the newly registered graduate nurse to treat them as partners and work with them to make a holistic and systematic assessment of their needs; to develop a personalised plan that is based on mutual understanding and respect for their individual situation promoting health and well-being, minimising risk of harm and promoting their safety at all times.

Entry to the register

12. In partnership with the person, their carers and their families, makes a holistic, person centred and systematic assessment of physical, emotional, psychological, social, cultural and spiritual needs, including risk, and together, develops a comprehensive personalised plan of nursing care.

Chapter aims

After reading this chapter you will be able to:

*   describe how the recovery approach can inform treatment and care in a variety of situations across the life span;
*   see how an understanding of our shared humanity can help you as a professional to engage with service users in a positive and creative manner;
*   consider the implications for people who access services but do not receive recovery-orientated services.

Introduction

The recovery approach has the potential to transform the delivery of not just mental health services but of all health care delivery across the life span and all health conditions, with people being active in and at the centre of their care, enabling then to take control over their own decisions and connect with their own communities. While there are some mental health services that have made important changes to how care is delivered, in the UK there are still significant challenges to how recovery-focused services are delivered. In particular, there is a lack of clear understanding of the concept of recovery and its practical application. Here, mental health nurses can be pivotal in developing recovery-focused care and support.

The recovery approach and its application have come under criticism for a number of reasons from various perspectives. There are professionals who argue that it can set unrealistic expectations for people, that it does not apply to people who are very unwell or are detained under the Mental Health Act or that it is nothing new and is something that is happening already. The survivor/consumer movement argue that it has been hijacked by clinicians (promoting a medicalised understanding of mental health) and health services and politicians (who use it to support neo-liberal ideas putting responsibility on individuals to become well and to justify the rationing of services).

This chapter will describe how understanding a person's social and political context can enable nurses to engage in recovery-orientated practice in a positive and creative way. It will explain and give examples of how the recovery approach can be used to support people in diverse contexts: from young people, people with long term conditions, people with dementia and older people. It will look at how a recovery approach can support service users to regain and maintain mental health.

Our recovery journey: shared humanity

It is not just the service users who use our services to whom the recovery principles apply. Often people are attracted to working in health care because of something they have experienced, or because of something experienced by a family member. Everyone at some stage in their lives faces traumatic and life-changing experiences. This may be having a mental health problem; the end of a relationship; the death or serious illness/injury of someone we love; losing a job or failing a key examination; being the victim of abuse or crime; being convicted of a crime; fleeing war or persecution and seeking asylum in another country. These are things that we 'recover' from, things that we have to learn to live with.

> *Because all people (helpers included) experience the catastrophes of life (death of a loved one, divorce, the threat of severe physical illness, and disability), the challenge of recovery must be faced. Successful recovery from a catastrophe does not change the fact that the experience has occurred, that the effects are still present, and that one's life has changed forever. Successful recovery does mean that the person has changed, and that the meaning of these facts to the person has therefore changed. They are no longer the primary focus of one's life. The person moves on to other interests and activities.*
> (Anthony, 1993, p17)

Clinical ideas about cure have no place in relation to such life challenges, and it is certainly not possible to 'turn the clock back' to the way things were before, but the challenge of recovery is very much present: accepting and overcoming what has happened and recovering a new sense of self and of purpose in our lives.

Activity 6.1   *Reflection*

Think back to a time when life was particularly difficult for you. What helped you get through it? What do you feel you learned from it? With the distance of time, in what way or ways do you think this period changed you?

If you found yourself in a similar situation now, would you react in the way that you did then, or has what you have learned changed your responses?

Understanding a shared humanity in the process of recovery can break down the 'us and them' between staff and people who use services and this can be key in building effective clinical relationships, whichever setting you are working in. Not only is recovery possible for everyone, the challenge of recovery is faced by everyone at some time in their lives.

However, while there may be a sense of a shared humanity, we also need to recognise people's experiences are different and, as we will come to discuss in this chapter, we cannot divorce the social and political context within which we live. Furthermore, unless we are aware of the stigma and discrimination that exists around mental ill-health, we will not appreciate the real issues in a person's life.

Recovery across the lifespan

If we understand recovery in this more personal and community-focused way, it makes the principles of recovery much more applicable to different contexts and a broader range of service areas. Though the word may not have the same resonance, the principles will be the same or similar. Ideas about recovery have primarily been explored in relation to people of working age. Even if the terminology is different, however, the underlying ideas are equally applicable to younger and older people, although the context of their journey might be different (DH, 2011).

> *Recovery is a personal process. Recovery is not always a cure. I think recovery is about how you try to tackle the bad effects of mental health problems. When things go wrong if we have hope we can change and develop and grow.*
> (Sadia, 14)
>
> *Recovery to me is being able to live around other people and not feel judged or compelled to behave a certain way. Recovery to me is being able to be who you really are without feeling ashamed or embarrassed ... you don't have to completely defeat your illness you just have to learn to live with it. And above all just remember that you DO matter and you ARE worth it!*
> (Nancy, 17)
>
> (Young people in a London adolescent unit cited by Perkins and Repper, 2015)

However, one young woman illustrated how the context of younger people's journeys may be different. She was worried about the idea of recovery as 'going back to how things were before':

> *Sometimes it can be a different experience to teenagers recovering than it is to adults. This is because teenagers are in a very different stage of life; they are still growing and developing, becoming the adults that they want to be. Whereas an adult may already be confident in who they are, a teenager is still discovering, exploring ... you may come out a different person to how they started off.*
> (Hannah, 15, cited in Perkins and Repper, 2015)

No-one, of course, can turn the clock back to how things were before. Everyone who is diagnosed with mental health problems faces the challenge of growing within and beyond what has happened to them. Everyone is 'growing and developing', 'exploring and discovering' ... and everyone comes out 'a different person to how they started off'.

> *You have the wondrously terrifying task of becoming who you are called to be. Your life and dreams may have been shattered – but from such ruins you can build a new life full of value and purpose.*
> (Deegan, 1993)

At the other end of the age spectrum, such a conception of recovery is equally relevant, although again the context may be somewhat different. Older people who experience mental health challenges often do this in the context of longer term physical health problems, loss of valued roles, the death of friends and loved ones and ageist assumptions about the value of their lives. Some may shy away from ideas about 'recovery' in relation to dementia because it gives 'false hope' of a 'cure', but, as Hill et al. (2010) describe, preferred terms may be less important than the values they support:

> *Even for conditions where there is as yet no cure, as with dementia, improvements in care and treatment are achievable ... 'Recovery' and well-being approaches ... are equally applicable to older people. 'Recovery' does not imply 'cure', but builds on the personal strengths and resilience of an individual ... Recovery is about the development of coping skills, and about social inclusion, making it possible for people to have quality of life and a degree of independence and choice, even those with the most enduring and disabling conditions.*
> (Social Care Institute of Excellence, 2006)

A diagnosis of dementia is certainly devastating and life changing, but many people living with the diagnosis and their families have shown that a decent life is possible.

> *You've got it, it's gonna kill you, but not today, so let's get on with it today and let's get today's enjoyment or whatever you like, and don't think about what's going to happen tomorrow or the next day. Live today. As I say although you've got it, it hasn't killed you so get on and enjoy.*
> (cited in Pratt and Wilkinson, 2001)
>
> *I'm living with Dementia, not dying from Dementia.*
> (Ashley, cited in Care Services Improvement Partnership, 2007)
>
> *The opportunity to 'continue to be me' is of the essence in living well with dementia.*
> (Daley et al., 2013)
>
> *I'm still me. My memory may not be as good as it was but it doesn't stop me from being me.*
> (cited in Care Services Improvement Partnership, 2007)

However, the opportunity to do this is often limited by attitudes. Nowhere are negative images more evident than in relation to those with a diagnosis of dementia, with popular ideas about 'living death', 'death that leaves the body behind' – and failure to provide the support people need to maintain both a sense of who they are and the activities they value.

> *Support is the key to me leading as normal a life as possible. People knowing and treating me as the person I still am. Giving me room to live.*
> (cited in Care Services Improvement Partnership, 2007)

There are also strong parallels with people who have physical disabilities. Ideas about recovery also have relevance beyond the mental health arena to people with acquired physical impairments and long-term health conditions. For people facing such challenges, ideas about 'cure' and 'going back to how things were before' are not relevant, but a recovery vision of 'living well with', 'recovering a new sense of self and of purpose within and beyond the limits of the disability' are equally pertinent. As long ago as 1988, Patricia Deegan drew parallels between physical and mental health challenges:

> *At a young age we had both experienced a catastrophic shattering of our world, hopes and dreams. He had broken his neck and was paralyzed and I was diagnosed as being schizophrenic ... Just days earlier we knew ourselves as young people with exciting futures, and then everything collapsed around us. As teenagers we were told that we would be 'sick' or 'disabled' for the rest of our lives.*
> (Deegan, 1988)

The process of 'discovering and exploring', 'growing and developing', 'becoming the adults that they want to be' is equally pertinent to everyone facing mental or physical health challenges. The benefit of an inclusive understanding of recovery is also the opportunity to break down the distinction between physical and mental health and offer a much more integrated approach.

Recovery-focused relationships in context

Most importantly, recovery (whatever our age or health condition) occurs within the context of relationships and it is in our relationships where hope is fostered, enabling us to explore our possibilities. It should be noted that social isolation is not only bad for mental health and wellbeing it is also important for physical health and is a major cause of premature death:

> *Social relationships, or the relative lack thereof, constitute a major risk factor for health – rivalling the effect of well-established health risk factors such as cigarette smoking, blood pressure, blood lipids, obesity and physical activity.*
> (House et al., 1988)

Often when people are cared for in services, they lose contact with their wider social connections and networks. People need to be assisted to find/maintain those ordinary, reciprocal relationships with friends and loved ones that are necessary to break out of this isolation that so often accompanies a diagnosis of mental health challenges. Relationships with mental health professionals can never replace partners, friends and neighbours, but they can nevertheless be particularly powerful ... for good or ill (Gilburt et al., 2008).

Trusting, empowering, hope-inspiring relationships are at the heart of recovery-focused services. But our relationships can also be barriers, such as when:

- One person talks about their thoughts and feelings, the other does not.

- One is in the role of helper and the other is in the role of being helped.

- One is there because they need help (or someone else thinks they need help), and the other is paid to be there.

- One person is 'the expert' who defines the others reality – has 'insight' into the real issues – and prescribes what is best for them (and, at the bottom line, can force them to adhere to these prescriptions via compulsory treatment).

All these barriers that divide 'them' from 'us' are compounded by our differences; in our culture, class, education, ethnicity, age, faith, belief and so forth. If we are truly to promote recovery, we must reach across the barriers that divide 'them' and 'us' and develop relationships that recognise and demonstrate our common humanity. We need to re-examine the traditional rules which assume that 'the expert knows best'. In recovery-focused services, there are two sets of expertise: professional expertise is based on research and clinical experience and the expertise of lived experience based on personal narratives. Developing relationships that break down 'them' and 'us' boundaries requires that we recognise the expertise of lived experience as well as professional expertise and bring these together in a process of genuine shared decision-making that really respects the person's preferences and experience (see Deegan and Drake, 2006). We as nurses bring three types of expertise to our work: our professional qualifications and experience, which includes our skills, talents, interests, beliefs, culture and so on; our experience of life; and our lived experience of trauma and recovery from trauma.

Research summary: Sharing experience to facilitate relationship building

Research conducted in Dorset found that people who have accessed services have found it helpful to their own recovery and wellbeing when staff have disclosed something of their own lived experience of past mental health challenges (Morgan and Lawson, 2015).

(continued)

(continued)

Morgan and Lawson (2015) also found that when staff using their own lived experience in this way:

- The 'them and us' perception is broken down, which in turn challenges stigma and discrimination.
- Opportunities are created to enhance practice, which gives a balanced understanding of academic expertise and lived experience expertise.
- Faith and belief in the efficiency of mental health services is increased.
- The experience for people who access services, their carers, supporters and staff is improved.
- Support for the wellbeing of staff is improved.
- A recovery-orientated ethos within services is promoted.

There can be no simple rules. We cannot replace the traditional 'tell nothing of yourself – be professional' rule with its opposite: treat this as an ordinary relationship and share whatever you want to share. These are not ordinary, everyday relationships – they are special, privileged relationships. Therefore, we need to move into that grey area in the middle: What should we share? When, how, why? We must always be guided by the purpose of our relationships – to assist people in their journey of recovery – and our own needs and sensitivities. For a discussion of these issues see Morgan and Lawson (2015).

Creating communities that accommodate recovery

Among people with a diagnosis of mental disorder (and/or physical or cognitive disorder), there are many challenges to live well and to rebuild meaningful, satisfying and contributing lives. To support this, we need to create communities that can accommodate all of us. There are two ways of thinking about inclusion and citizenship. First, there is the clinical model typically adopted by mental health services that focuses on changing the person so they fit in (via treatment/therapy, skills training etc.). But there is also a social model and human rights framework adopted by the broader disability movement which focuses not on changing the person but on changing the world so that it can accommodate everyone.

Activity 6.2   *Critical thinking*

To find one social and human rights framework, go to:

www.copower.org/models-of-disability/179-rights-based-model-of-disability.html

Here you will find two definitions of a social disability rights model from the Michigan Disability Rights Coalition.

After reading through the two definitions and making notes, consider the following questions:

- Which of the two definitions speaks most deeply to you?
- What modifications (if any) might need to be made to your preferred definition to make it fully applicable to a UK context?

If we are to effectively promote the recovery approach within services we need to think differently about the way we understand the challenges people face and the support we provide (Perkins, 2012; Repper and Perkins, 2012). If we use a human rights and social model it will do three things. First, it requires that we move away from asking 'what is wrong with the person' and 'how can we put it right' to asking:

- What are the barriers that prevent participation?
- What supports and adjustments would the person like to get around these barriers to do the things they want to do and live the life they want to lead? What are the mental health equivalents of the wheelchair, hearing loop, the lift, the personal assistant, sign language interpreter etc.?
- How can we enable people to understand and assert their rights to participation and inclusion?

Second, it requires that we recognise the resources available within communities. Helping people to access opportunities they value and participate as equal citizens (in families/intimate relationships, workplaces, colleges, faith communities, social and leisure activities) is about supporting a relationship. If people are to access opportunities, they value it may be necessary to provide support not only to individuals but also to people and organisations within those communities. This 'social model' focuses on barriers because it argues that:

> *It is society that disables people. It is attitudes, actions, assumptions – social, cultural and physical structures which disable by erecting barriers and imposing restrictions and options. Disability is not inherent ... The social model of disability is about nothing more complicated than a clear focus on the economic, environmental and cultural barriers encountered by people who are viewed by others as having some form of impairment – whether physical, sensory or intellectual.*
> (Oliver, 2004)

While recognising differences in nature and context, among the originators of ideas about recovery, recognition of the parallels between the challenges faced by people diagnosed with mental health issues and those faced by people living with physical/sensory impairments and other long-term health conditions has long been recognised:

> *For most of us, mental health problems are a given ... the real problems exist in the form of barriers in the environment that prevent us from living, working and learning in environments of our choice. [The task is] to confront, challenge and change those barriers and to make environments*

accessible … environments are not just physical places but also social and interpersonal environments … those of us with psychiatric disabilities face many environmental barriers that impede and thwart our efforts to live independently and gain control over our lives.
(Deegan, 1992)

It is a social model of disability that underpins the UN Convention on the Rights of Persons with Disabilities (2006) which includes people with a diagnosis of mental health problems as well as those with other long-term or recurring health conditions, physical/sensory impairments and learning disabilities. Ratified by the UK and 227 other countries, this convention starts from the premise of moving away from

viewing persons with disabilities as 'objects' of charity, medical treatment and social protection towards viewing persons with disabilities as 'subjects' with rights, who are capable of claiming those rights and making decisions for their lives based on their free and informed consent as well as being active members of society.
(UN Convention on the Rights of Persons with Disabilities, 2006)

This includes the right to both the same rights and opportunities as other citizens (at home, at work and as members of the community) and the right to the support and adjustments (based on their own preferences and choices) needed to participate as equal citizens in all facets of economic, social and community life.

Inclusion and citizenship are not about 'becoming normal' but creating inclusive communities that can accommodate all of us. Not about 'becoming independent' but having the right to support and adjustments (in line with our choices and aspirations) to ensure full and equal participation and citizenship.
(Slade et al., 2014)

Case study

Jane had always wanted to go to college, but she found it difficult because on some days she could not get out of the house and she was very anxious about going into a room full of people on her own. She also dreaded the tutor 'picking on her': asking her questions in front of the class. In conversation with Jane, it transpired that she had a friend (Anya, a fellow inpatient she had met while on the ward) who also wanted to go to the college. Therefore, it was agreed that Anya would call round to Jane's flat on her way to college so that they could go in together. This provided the extra support that Jane needed to get to college, although there were also times when, even with support, she could not make it out of her flat and could not bear to sit in the room full of students for the whole session. Therefore, her care co-ordinator arranged for Jane, Anya and their tutor to meet, discuss Jane's problems with anxiety and work out ways around them. A number of adjustments were agreed that Jane felt would enable her to take the course:

- *If she was unable to get to class, the tutor would send the materials and exercises home for her (either in the post or give them to Anya to drop them off).*
- *If she felt unable to stay in the class, it would be OK for her to leave and go and sit quietly in the library (if this happened then the tutor would take her the work she had missed so she could catch up).*
- *The tutor would not ask her questions: only if she put her hand up and indicated that she wanted to say something would the tutor call on her.*

In order to support the tutor, the care co-ordinator gave her his mobile number and said she could call if she was concerned.

Third, we must not only think about the **community** as being the geographical community where people live. We must also think about:

- Communities of identification: people who the person sees as being like them for example, helping someone to access a particular faith community or lesbian/gay community.
- Communities of interest: people who share interests with the person, for example, political parties, sporting or arts activities.
- E-communities and opportunities: the internet contains a wealth of information and possibilities for contact, and e-exclusion simply compounds the exclusion that is so often a consequence of mental health challenges thus rendering the person further isolated and alone.
- Peer communities: peer-led groups and organisations as well as individuals within the person's network who share similar challenges.

In all of these areas, assistance might involve helping the person discover what is out there (groups – real or virtual – literature etc.) and working with them to organise the support and adjustments that they may need to avail themselves of these opportunities (someone to assist them to get there, internet access etc.).

Finally, and most importantly, we must make sure that people are aware of their rights, especially their rights under the 2010 Equality Act, and know how to exert these rights.

People with mental health conditions are covered by the disability rights provisions within this Act which not only outlaw discrimination but also require that employers, education providers and all providers of goods and services (from the health service to the gym and local shops) make 'reasonable adjustments' to facilitate access. In the above example, the adjustments made to enable Jane to access the course she wanted to study would all qualify as 'reasonable adjustments'.

It is also important that we tell people what they can do if they feel that they have experienced discrimination or been denied the adjustments they need. Clearly, mental health workers cannot be legal experts, but they can help people to access the support they need. There is also a free national Equality Advisory Support Service and locally there may be Legal Advice Centres and Citizens Advice Bureaux who can help.

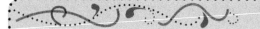

Chapter summary

By looking at the importance of recovery no matter what stage of life a person is at, this chapter has explored the importance of services that engage with people in their own contexts, of community, family and lifestyle. This approach also encourages us to think about our own journeys of recovery, how we relate to service users, and how recovery principles can be applied across a range of health conditions and with different age groups.

Promoting recovery for people who are being cared for within health care services (a hospital, a secure mental health unit or even a prison) is discussed in more detail in Chapter 7.

Further reading

Allen, S. (2010) *Our stories: Moving on. Recovery and well-being.* London: South West London and St. George's Mental Health NHS Trust.

Repper, J. and Perkins, R. (2003) *Social inclusion and recovery.* London: Bailliere Tindall.

Useful websites

www.england.nhs.uk/mentalhealth/ NHS England.

www.hscic.gov.uk/mentalhealth Health and Social Care Information Centre (HSCIC).

Chapter 7
Creating recovery-focused services

Rachel Perkins and Phil Morgan

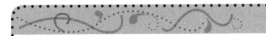

NMC Standards for Pre-registration Nursing Education

Domain 1: Professional values

4. All nurses must work in partnership with service users, carers, families, groups, communities and organisations. They must manage risk, and promote health and wellbeing while aiming to empower choices that promote self-care and safety.

4.1. **Mental health nurses** must work with people in a way that values, respects and explores the meaning of their individual lived experiences of mental health problems, to provide person-centred and recovery-focused practice.

Domain 2: Communication and interpersonal skills

5. All nurses must use therapeutic principles to engage, maintain and, where appropriate, disengage from professional caring relationships, and must always respect professional boundaries.

Domain 3: Nursing practice and decision-making

3. All nurses must carry out comprehensive, systematic nursing assessments that take account of relevant physical, social, cultural, psychological, spiritual, genetic and environmental factors, in partnership with service users and others through interaction, observation and measurement.

Domain 4: Leadership, management and team working

4. All nurses must be self-aware and recognise how their own values, principles and assumptions may affect their practice. They must maintain their own personal and professional development, learning from experience, through supervision, feedback, reflection and evaluation.

Essential Skills Clusters

Care, compassion and communication

5. People can trust the newly registered graduate nurse to engage with them in a warm, sensitive and compassionate way.

(continued)

continued . . . •••

6. People can trust the newly registered graduate nurse to engage therapeutically and actively listen to their needs and concerns, responding using skills that are helpful, providing information that is clear, accurate, meaningful and free from jargon.

Entry to the register

13. Uses appropriate and relevant communication skills to deal with difficult and challenging circumstances, for example, responding to emergencies, unexpected occurrences, saying 'no', dealing with complaints, resolving disputes, de-escalating aggression, conveying 'unwelcome news'.

Chapter aims

After reading this chapter you should be able to:

-   describe how the recovery approach can inform treatment and care across a range of mental health settings, including secure units and units where people are compulsorily detained;
-   understand the importance of using your own lived experience within the context of a therapeutic relationship;
-   help service users to become more independent and self-confident in preparation for a return to, and living well, in the community.

Introduction

In the previous chapter, we spent some time thinking about recovery across and throughout our lives. In this chapter we consider how we can utilise recovery-focused approaches to create inspiring health care environments for service users and staff. The *Safewards Initiative*, for example, was designed to explore ways of increasing safety on inpatient wards and reducing coercion by promoting better relationships between staff and patients (Bowers et al., 2014). One of the effective ways for achieving this involved staff disclosing non-controversial information about themselves:

> *If [service users can be] given a little more information about us, they can find areas of common interest and conversational topics. The mutual familiarity and knowledge gleaned can help the faster forming of relationships. And those relationships can help us orientate patients, enhance their coping skills, ameliorate their more difficult behaviour and make them feel more comfortable and reassured during their admission.*
> (Safewards, 2016)

However, as discussed in Chapter 6, nurses may have lived experience of trauma and many have also themselves experienced mental distress and mental health challenges. This too is important information that can be used to enhance relationships and better promote recovery.

Creating recovery-focused services

As we discussed in Chapter 6, not only do communities need to accommodate recovery, health care services also need to consider what they can do to better facilitate recovery. The implications are that mental health services need to reposition their focus from a more dominant clinical approach to one that enhances or enables personal recovery. Central to this is valuing and learning from the lived experience of people using these services, along with their carers and supporters.

While services cannot 'do' recovery, or 'recover' people, they can support or hinder people in their journey (O'Hagan, 2014). Everyone's recovery journey is unique and deeply personal (Anthony, 1993), but the accounts of people who have rebuilt their lives with a diagnosis of mental ill-health challenges strongly suggests that three things are particularly important (Repper and Perkins, 2003, 2012; Shepherd et al., 2008; Perkins, 2012):

1   Hope. It is not possible to rebuild your life unless you believe that a decent life is possible and you need people around who believe in your possibilities.

2   Control and self-determination. Taking back control over your destiny, the challenges you face and the help you receive to overcome them.

3   Opportunity and participation. The chance to do the things that you value, access those opportunities that all citizens should expect and participate in society as an equal citizen.

This experiential expertise is supported by empirical research. In his extensive review of the international research literature Warner (2009) demonstrates three things to be important in recovery: optimism, empowerment and employment.

The question we have to ask ourselves is whether we have created hopeful, empowering environments that enable people to discover their possibilities and pursue their ambitions.

> *[W]e are learning that the environment around people must change if we are to be expected to grow into the fullness of the person who, like a small seed, is waiting to emerge from within each of us ... How do we create hope filled, humanized environments and relationships in which people can grow?*
> (Deegan, 1996)

Too often people experience mental health services eroding hope, taking control over their lives and failing to assist them in pursuing their dreams and ambitions (O'Hagan, 2014).

In creating recovery-focused services, the first challenge is to understand what the world looks like from the perspective of the individual and the context of their life. Services need to recognise that people are the experts in determining their own requirements and can play an active role in meeting their own needs, rather than being passive dependents/recipients of the ministrations of professionals. While appreciating the devastating impact of what has happened and being with the person in their anger and distress, nurses must also foster hope and images of possibility. The challenge is for professionals to move from being 'on top' to being 'on tap' (Repper and Perkins, 2003; Perkins, 2012) – supporting self-management and putting their expertise at the disposal of those who require it rather than telling them what to do, and enabling people to explore what is important to them and pursue their ambitions and dreams.

Creating more recovery-focused services is not an 'add on' to existing ways of doing things – a new service, new workers, new interventions – but requires a fundamental change in philosophy, culture and practice (Shepherd et al., 2008; Perkins, 2012). It requires that we consider everything that we do (from giving out medication in hospital through providing information and practical assistance, to the individual conversations and 'one to one' sessions that we have) through the lens of recovery.

Activity 7.1   *Reflection*

Think about a service user you encountered who was at a point in the journey of recovery. Consider your own relationship with this person and reflect upon the following questions:

Did I try to understand the situation from the person's perspective?

Did I foster hope and images of possibility?

Did I enable the person to take back control over their life, problems and help they receive?

Did I help the person to do the things they value and participate in the communities of their choice? (See, for example, Shepherd et al., 2008, '10 top tips' for recovery-orientated practice.)

You might want to talk with your mentor about any issues this activity has raised for you.

Recovery-focused practice in inpatient settings

There are many services whose culture remains rooted in less forward-looking models of care. In part this can be a distortion of the culture of risk- assessment, where the risks to be assessed are all seen in a negative light, as threats ... Such wards ... may be holding back patients' recovery ... Values such as respect, choice, patient involvement and autonomy should be seen as integral to all aspects of psychiatric care, rather than being only a counterbalance to its more coercive aspects. (Mental Health Act Commission, 2009)

It is clearly important to consider the role of recovery within people's own communities. For many people, however, the experience of mental health services includes admissions to inpatient services. Too often, admission to hospital is seen as a 'failure' of community services or a 'failure' of the individual to comply with the prescriptions of the experts. This is a mistake. First, many mental health conditions fluctuate, with or without treatment and therapy, therefore the challenge is how to minimise the impact of these fluctuations on a person's life. Second, when a person is very distressed then home may not be the best place to be. It is difficult for a partner or a child to see their partner/mother in a very distressed state and unable to do the things they can usually do, and it can be very difficult to be around someone who is in crisis. Often the best way of preserving important relationships is a period of respite – relief from day to day responsibilities until the crisis abates.

Crises and set-backs are part of life and part of the recovery process. The challenge is to learn from these and grow stronger because of them. This means that acute inpatient admission can be a very important part of a person's recovery journey – for good or ill. Too often acute admission wards are not seen or experienced as the safe 'retreat' where people can grow and regain their strength, but have taken on a more custodial role.

> *All staff time and resources are spent to stop bad things happening but not make good things happen.*
> (Mind, 2011)

If inpatient wards are to assist people in their recovery journey, it is critical that they foster hope, promote personal control and self-determination, and enable people to access the opportunities that they value.

In forensic services, the challenges are often bigger challenges and restrictions greater. People admitted to high or medium secure services not only have to find ways of growing within and beyond a diagnosis of mental health challenges, they also face the task of accommodating and moving beyond the things they have done and the crimes they have committed. They can also expect to spend a considerable length of time in a secure setting deprived of many freedoms they have hitherto enjoyed.

However, different service contexts create different challenges and possibilities. Much consideration of recovery has focused on community services – relatively less attention has been paid to crisis and inpatient settings. The complexity is particularly challenging when people are compulsorily detained under the Mental Health Act.

Recovery-focused practice in the context of compulsory detention

As ideas of recovery have become popular, rates of compulsory detention and treatment in the UK have risen alarmingly. In 1997/8 there were 38,695 detentions; a decade later this had risen to 44,093 detentions. In 2008 **Community Treatment Orders** (CTO) were introduced. It was argued that these would reduce the need for compulsory hospitalisation, but the number of compulsory detentions has continued to rise. By 2013/14 the number of detentions had risen to 53,176 (Care Quality Commission, 2014) and an additional 5365 people were being treated on CTOs. By 2012/13 CTO powers had been used 18,942 times (Care Quality Commission, 2013) rising from 2134 in 2008/9 to 4647 in 2013/14. It should be noted that both a systematic review of the literature (Kisely et al., 2011) and a randomised controlled trial in the UK (Burns et al., 2013) found that CTOs were ineffective in reducing hospitalisation or improving clinical or social functioning.

Many have argued that compulsory detention and treatment are antithetical to recovery:

> *The recovery philosophy's cornerstones of self-determination, connection to our communities, social justice and a broad choice of services are a direct challenge to the use of compulsory interventions, particularly if they are not applied on an equal basis with other citizens.*
> (O'Hagan, 2014)

> *Participants identified that the main barrier to the formation of a therapeutic relationship was the experience of coercion. Relationships that were perceived as coercive were always described as negative and resulted in negative patient experiences.*
> (Gilburt et al., 2008)

> *[I]t works against the recovery goal of reclaiming a meaningful life – a process that is based on self- determination and respect for the individual as a citizen of society.*
> (Slade et al., 2014)

However, it remains the case that nurses and other health care professionals practise in the context of compulsory detention and those who are detained still face the challenge of recovery. To promote recovery-focused practice in the context of compulsory detention, it is therefore incumbent on practitioners to do the following.

- Reduce the need to use compulsory detention by, for example, planning for crises which can also significantly reduce compulsory detention. Henderson et al. (2004) describes the co-production of a joint crisis plan which 'is developed by seeking agreement between the patient and their mental health team about what to do if they become unwell in the future ... [and] can include things like an individual the patient would like to have contacted in a crisis; treatments that have been helpful or unhelpful in the past; treatment preferences or refusals, and practical arrangements'. Research shows that such joint crisis plans can significantly reduce rates of compulsory detention (Henderson et al., 2004): at 15-month follow-up 13% of those who had a joint crisis plan and 27% of those who did not had been compulsorily detained.

- Do our best to ensure that people have a positive experience: little acts of kindness can go a long way. For example, making someone a cup of tea when they are very distressed, or ensuring that someone has access to their favourite book or music or food (Gilburt et al., 2008).

- Minimise the extent to which compulsory detention impedes a person's recovery. As Roberts et al. (2008) have argued, there should be no 'recovery free' zones within services. While hospital admission may decrease some risks, it also increases others, for example:

  o Loss of hope.

  o Loss of self-determination and self-control.

  o Loss of belief that you can be the author of your own destiny.

  o Loss of friends and social contacts.

  o Loss of valued social roles.

  o Loss of college place, work and so on.

All of these are of critical importance in recovery, therefore mitigating these risks in relation to recovery is central. Roberts et al. (2008) suggest that

> *the therapeutic purpose of detaining someone and treating them against their will is to achieve the gradual handing back of choice and control in ways that are safe and to enable them to resume responsibility for themselves.*

- Develop a different approach to risk: from managing risk to promoting safety and opportunity in the context of co-produced safety plans.

> *Service users expressed concern at the lack of attention to their wider social care needs … particularly when the focus has been on problems and risk … rather than building on their strengths towards recovery.*
> (DH, 2006b)

> *[P]sychiatrists … reported that risk was dominating their practice … which was having a damaging impact on their clinical practice, undermining meaningful clinical decision making and making engagement with patients more difficult.*
> (Royal College of Psychiatrists, 2008)

Humanising care and creating hope-inspiring services

In both acute admission wards and longer term or forensic settings, it is critical that we think about the way we welcome people when they arrive, how we allay their fears, and sympathise with their anger and hopelessness about being admitted. The environment of the ward is central to fostering hope and humanising care – what sort of messages does it convey about the possibilities for life with mental health challenges (images, recovery stories) and the value (or lack of it) of the people within it (separate 'staff' and 'patient' toilets, crockery etc.)?

For in-patient nursing staff, admissions are a regular occurrence – part of the day to day routine – but for each person who is admitted, even if they have been on the ward before, this is typically a frightening and/or devastating life event.

> *When I first went in I felt hopeless, I was lost … I thought it was the end of my world.*
> (Young man talking about his admission to a forensic unit in Allen, 2010)
>
> *They are all very nice to me here but I don't think they understand what a big deal this is for me. Last week I was a mother walking down the road with her children in a buggy – now I'm just a mental patient.*
> (Woman on an acute admission ward in south London)

In order to understand where the person is coming from, we must explore how the person feels about being in hospital – what it means to them – as well as any concerns or fears they have about being there: both things outside hospital (is my house secure, who will look after the cat, will my friends ever speak to me again, I will never be able to be a mother or get a decent job now etc.) and things within the hospital (fears for personal safety, not knowing what will happen etc.).

Listening to personal narratives

Narratives are central to recovery. People may feel that no-one listens to their side of things – offering to put their account, in their words, in the clinical records can both help the person to feel heard and others to understand where they are coming from. Instead of starting with our standard assessments and checklists, it is often best to start with a cup of tea and the person's own story about what has happened: 'I guess you must have had a bad time, what has happened to bring you here?' Rather than challenging aspects of the person's narrative it is important to be empathic: there is always more than one way of looking at things and the person's own perspective (not just that of their parents, the police, mental health professionals) is critical and can offer a much richer account of their experience.

This is well illustrated by O'Hagan (1996) where she presents the entries in her diary during in an admission to hospital alongside those in the clinical notes. For example, Figure 7.1 contrasts the psychiatric notes from the day of her admission with her diary entry for the same day.

Entry in psychiatric notes	Mary's own diary entry
Mary is a 25-year-old Caucasian university student who has a history of manic depressive psychosis. Now appears to be entering a depressive phase. Quiet and withdrawn. Dresses unconventionally. Not an easy patient to relate to. She plays her cards very close to her chest.	*Today I went to see the psychiatrist. He is a little man with a beard and glasses and he wrote his notes in small, tidy handwriting. He stared right through me. I kept thinking he could see into every corner of my mind. Every time I moved – the way I sat, where I put my hands – I thought would be used as evidence of my badly diseased mind. I was afraid he had the power to trick me into letting out my biggest secrets. I was too terrified to talk to him.*

Figure 7.1: Contrasting perspectives: psychiatric notes and service user diary entry

As a person moves forward, narratives can be important in understanding and celebrating progress. Many people have found keeping a diary to be important in helping them through difficult times in their life. A diary can:

- Help you to face up to what has happened.
- Reaffirm your experiences.
- Help you to reflect and clarify your thoughts.
- Help you to make sense of what is happening.
- Help you to explore yourself and your experience of the world.
- Help you to see the progress you have made.
- Provide comfort during challenging periods.

Peer support

Peer support can be really important in offering hope, imagining possibilities and helping people to find the courage they need to keep going when they are unable to see any light at the end of the tunnel.

> *I ... benefited from speaking to others with mental health problems. I got more 'therapy' from them than I did any of the staff.*
> (Mind, 2011)

There are many ways of offering peer support including collecting and making available recovery stories. Some wards have started collecting the recovery stories of people who have left the ward/hospital and moved on in their lives, informal conversations with others on the ward, people who have been on the ward coming back and talking about their experiences, inviting self-help groups/peers to run sessions on the ward (e.g. 'hearing voices groups') and by employing peer support workers as part of the staff team (see Repper et al., 2013a and 2013b). Peer support has also been extended to prisons. The majority of prisons in England and Wales now have a Samaritan-supported 'Listener' scheme. Listeners, who work as unpaid volunteers, provide confidential emotional support to other prisoners. 'Insiders' are selected prisoner volunteers who are trained volunteers to provide basic information and reassurance to prisoners new to prison shortly after their arrival in prison.

Sometimes peer support can be very informal.

Case study

Hayley – with a 10-year-old child (who was doing very well at school and at home) – was admitted to an inpatient ward and was terrified that her child would be taken into care. A member of staff knew another woman – Anne – who had mental health challenges and was successfully raising a child. She arranged for Anne to come in and talk to Hayley. Meeting someone else who had faced similar challenges helped Hayley to see how she would be able to look after her child and prepared her for the assessments and challenges that might lie ahead. Anne has since gone on, with the help of the staff member, to set up a support group for mothers with mental health challenges.

Supporting the personal search for meaning

Devastating and life-changing events cause most people to ask some of those big questions about the meaning of life: 'Why?', 'Why me?', What now?', 'What's the point?', 'Who am I?'

> *When all you can see is the ward and those surroundings it is hard, but there is something to aspire to and work towards. ... it is good to have some kind of faith, not necessarily God, but some kind of higher force, something you can live for.*
> (in Allen, 2010)

For many people, the quest for meaning lies not in psychiatry but in spirituality or philosophy: having the opportunity to reflect on the ideas they value, the experiences that have shaped their life, what matters to them and what is important to them. An acute crisis offers a space to think and reflect on life as does a longer stay in a forensic setting which makes such reflection very important.

Changing our language

The language that we use is also important in creating a hope-inspiring environment. Too often the language of mental health focuses on what is wrong, not what is strong: narratives of deficit, dysfunctions, problems and fading life chances.

> [E]ven the briefest perusal of the current literature on schizophrenia will immediately reveal ... that this collection of problems is viewed by practitioners almost exclusively in terms of dysfunction and disorder. A positive or charitable phrase or sentence rarely meets the eye.

> [D]eficit-obsessed research can only produce theories and attitudes that are disrespectful of clients and are also likely to induce behaviour in clinicians such that service users are not listened to properly, treated as inadequate and ... not expected to become independent or competent individuals.
> (Chadwick, 1997)

The foundations for recovery and growing do not lie in a person's problems, deficits and dysfunctions but in their strengths, interests and resources. Language matters because language and thought are intimately interrelated: the way we speak and write about people determines the way we think about them. There is much in the psychiatric lexicon that is pejorative and focuses on what is wrong rather than what is strong. There is little hope-inspiring about language like 'non-compliant', 'attention-seeking', 'schizophrenic', 'lacking motivation', 'manipulative'. The alternatives may take more words, but they also offer greater possibilities: 'knows his own mind', 'recognises she needs help and values our help', 'person living with a diagnosis of schizophrenia', 'we have not yet found what drives him/what interests him', 'trying to get the help he needs' ... The term 'manipulative' is an interesting one: if a nurse is able to persuade a service user to do what he thinks is best, he is a good clinician, but if a person using services tries to get services to do what he thinks is best he is manipulative!

The language we use also needs to foster choice and control. Much of our language is quite prescriptive: 'You should ...', 'You must ...', 'My advice to you is ...', 'The best thing for you to do is ...'. On the other hand, large open-ended questions like 'what do you want?' are often very difficult to answer, especially if someone is very distressed or has become accustomed to be told what to do in services for a very long time. Instead, we can help people to exert some control by offering a range of options as suggestions. For example, 'Some people have found X helpful, some people have found Y helpful, some people have found Z helpful. Have you had any thoughts about what might help you?' It is important that choice extends beyond the options for help to the way in which people understand their problems. Instead of routinely providing the usual 'bio-psycho-social' models of mental health challenges, we could present people with the range of theories about mental health problems and let them make up their own mind which makes sense to them.

Activity 7.2 — Communication

We can broadly categorise the language we use when speaking to service users in terms of the following grid.

	Encouraging	Neutral	Discouraging	Stigmatising
Statement				
Description				
Open question				
Closed question				

Now look at the following phrases and decide where on the grid each one fits best.

- He will never be able to do that!
- Would you like me to help you?
- A 36-year-old gentleman.
- You never learn, do you?
- A man who is working towards turning his life around.
- What could he achieve given his unreliability?
- He has not achieved much in his life.
- That's great! Well done!
- What can I do to help you?
- You have tried this before and failed, haven't you?
- Drug addicts are always unreliable.
- Well, what do you expect from him?
- He has two children who he visits regularly.
- How are you?
- He is a drug addict.
- Do you have children?

An answer to this activity is given at the end of the chapter.

Fostering self-determination

Even if someone is compulsorily detained there is much that we can do to offer choice and help them to have some control over their life, their problems and the help they receive. There is much choice that can be offered within the limits of detention, for example, what time you want to get up in the morning, when you would like your leave and how you would like to use it, which of the activities/therapies on the ward you would like to do, other things you could do if none of these appeal to you, how you occupy your time, how you want to use your session's professionals, how you want to use (and what you want to ask at) your review meetings.

Helping people to start thinking about plans for looking after themselves and keeping themselves well can also be important: a crisis offers a valuable learning opportunity. In an inpatient setting people can start developing their own Personal Recovery Plans or 'Wellness Recovery Action Plans': things the person can do to keep themselves well, manage their ups and downs and cope with the vicissitudes of life. This may involve a number of areas, as outlined in Figure 7.2.

What to include	Comments and examples	Service user notes
Things to do every day or week to keep yourself on an even keel (sometimes called a 'daily maintenance plan').	This might include chores and responsibilities, but it should also include treats like having a long hot bath, watching your favourite TV programme, a cup of hot chocolate before bed.	I need to keep on top of my regular responsibilities. I enjoy a daily walk.
A 'first aid kit' of things you can do when you feel upset, worried, stressed, angry, disappointed, frustrated.	Many people have a first aid kit for minor cuts and bruises of the body (sticking plaster, bandages, antiseptic cream etc.) but people also need a first aid kit for bodily cuts and bruises for mental/emotional cuts and bruises. Different people find different things helpful: listening to music, going for a walk, having a cup of tea, talking to a friend, remembering something you like, looking forward to something that will happen, writing it all down.	When I am really stressed, I like to eat a marmite sandwich or take a walk. It's best I avoid other people when I am upset as I tend to have a go at them, even if it isn't their fault. Also best to avoid drinking alcohol.
Identifying the things that get to you – upset, worry, stress, anger, disappoint, frustrate you – and what you can do to stop them getting to you too much.	For example, painful anniversaries or times of year, someone putting us down, people not doing what they say they will do … It may be possible to avoid some things, but it is inevitable that things will happen that upset us, so plans for looking after ourselves are important. Often there are things in your 'first aid kit' that may be helpful.	I really don't like the short, dark days of winter.
Identifying signs that you are having a bad day and what you can do to look after yourself and get back on an even keel.	Sometimes these are called 'early warning signs' but they may just be the ordinary ups and downs that everyone experiences. They may be thoughts, feelings or behaviours that tell you all is not well.	
Identifying when everything is getting too much and what you can do to stop things getting worse – get back on an even keel.	Try to keep a mental note of signs that, for you, mean a crisis is looming.	

Figure 7.2: Template for a Personal Recovery Plan

Some people may not feel able or willing to write out formal plans, so it may be necessary to help people to think about things gradually: if a person has had a bad day, discussions of what has happened to upset them and what might make them feel better can be the starting point. Often, in inpatient settings, workshops where people can think about some of these things in a group setting can be helpful; often people get ideas from each other. Making it clear that such plans are ordinary – useful for everyone – not something special for those with mental health challenges can be important. In this context it is useful if staff share their own 'first aid kits', the things that get to them etc. Indeed, many staff have found it helpful to develop their own 'health and well-being at work' plans using these headings (see Perkins, 2013, *Surviving and Thriving at Work*).

Sharing decision-making and creating opportunities for participation in care

As well as genuine shared decision-making in relation to treatment and support planning (Deegan and Drake, 2006; Deegan, 2007, Deegan et al., 2008; US Department of Health and Human Services, Substance Abuse and Mental Health Services Administration, 2011) other ways of fostering control and self-determination include shared entries and self-help notes. Instead of writing progress and session notes about people, write notes with people and include both perspectives if the person and staff member disagree and give the person a copy so that they have a record of what has happened and what has been agreed.

Help people to develop ways of monitoring their own ups and downs. Instead of staff 'monitoring mental state' people can be assisted to monitor their own ups and downs, for example on a simple 'traffic light' system (green – what I am like when things are going OK; amber = early warning signs; red = signs that a crisis is looming) or a more sophisticated scale from 'what things are like at their worst' to 'what things are like when I am OK'. Sometimes this may need to be in terms of the person's own perceptions, for example, if a person believes the television is controlling their thoughts, the intensity of control may be recorded.

Maintaining social contacts and relationships

Too often, when people are in inpatient settings, they progressively lose more and more roles and relationships outside until the only role they have left is that of 'mental patient' and the only relationships they have are with mental health services. It is therefore important to maintain valued social roles and relationships during the inpatient stay/crisis.

To start off with, this might involve many things, for example:

- Letting friends, family and neighbours (anyone who is important to the person) know what has happened. There are many ways of doing this (a letter, a phone call, an e-mail, a text message ...) and the person can give as much or as little detail as they choose – maybe just saying that they are not well and will get in touch when they feel better.
- Cancelling appointments/engagements.
- A sick note to an employer or college.
- Helping the person to make arrangements for covering their day to day responsibilities.

Once immediate arrangements like this have been made, it is important to think about how to maintain relationships with people who are important to the person (including employers, colleges etc.) during the course of the admission. This may involve helping those who are important to the person to understand and accommodate what has happened and helping the individual to think about whether/what/when/how they will talk about the mental health challenges they have faced.

The next step is then to help people to resume their roles and relationships as soon as they can – this process can start while the person is still an inpatient. This may involve:

- Making apologies – sometimes people have not always behaved in ways that they are proud of while they have been in crisis – and saying thank you to people who have helped them. Sometimes people prefer to do this in the form of a letter, a phone call, an e-mail, a text message rather than a face to face meeting.

- Sorting out problems caused by the crisis/admission to hospital, for example, helping the person to sort out their flat, or debts.

- Making a plan to gradually resume relationships and activities and the help they will need.

- Deciding what to tell people.

Case study

Miles, a young man in an acute unit, is recovering well except for continuing anxiety. A sympathetic nurse encourages him to open up about anything that might be bothering him and discovers that he feels he behaved very badly to his gran shortly before admission. He shouted at her and broke one of her ornaments. He feels very guilty about this and this is preoccupying him at the moment.

The nurse, Jamil, encourages him to write an apology to his gran. He offers to help Miles choose a nice card from the hospital shop and suggests that once he is discharged and back at work he might like to draw up a savings plan so that he can save enough money to buy another ornament for her.

A period in hospital can offer opportunities to discover new possibilities: to take stock of life, work out what you have gained from your journey, work out what is important to you and, if necessary, change direction in life and embark on new possibilities. This is particularly important for people who may be in forensic inpatient facilities for many years.

> *I lost vital years of my life locked up, some dreams went out of the window ... but I feel stronger than ever now ... and wiser. ... I am content. I'm very into my music and performing, making tracks, writing poetry. I am graduating this year from an Open University degree. I've passed my driving test. I have a car.*
> (A man who had spent many years in a secure hospital, in Allen, 2010)

In longer-term inpatient settings this may involve:

- Rebuilding your life within the hospital environment. The chance to contribute within the ward/hospital: work and doing things for others enables people to start seeing themselves as more than a 'mental patient'.

> *I got involved in the work schemes on offer such as working in the library ... it was good to have a purpose and something to do.*
> (See Allen, 2010)

- Preparing for life outside the hospital: work, education, training as a bridge to the community.

> *I did courses ... Towards the end of my time [in hospital] I was able to get involved in some voluntary work helping at a daycentre for the elderly. This was good and it also built up my CV.*
> (See Allen, 2010)

Redefining risk and co-produced safety plans

Developing a recovery-focused approach to risk and safety is central to the development of more recovery-focused practice (see Perkins and Goddard, 2008; Boardman and Roberts, 2014; Perkins and Repper, 2016). While recovery involves taking some risks, safety is important. A recovery-focused approach to risk must bring together the expertise of lived experience and professional expertise and be founded on a shared understanding, shared decision-making and shared responsibility for safety. A person's behaviour is determined by their understanding of the situation and the things that are important to them: behaviour is only 'unpredictable' if we do not know how things look from the person's perspective. Maximising safety requires that we understand the context of the behaviour from the person's perspective.

> *The recovery ... philosophy requires the professional to be curious about what drives the service-user, what is meaningful to him, and why.*
> (Scott Moncrieff et al., 2009: An independent investigation into the care and treatment of Daniel Gonzales)

People may have very different understandings of things that have happened in the past ('risk history') to that recorded in their notes. For example, the risk history for one woman said she was a fire risk, having set fire to her kitchen. Her account was that she had left a frying pan on the hob when she went to answer a knock on the door, and although the pan was alight when she came back, she had put it out successfully and there was no damage to her kitchen. Understanding and recording the person's perspective as well can be really important in both increasing staff understanding or risk and safety and improving relationships by helping the person to feel heard and understood.

Case study

Individuals and professionals often have different perspectives on risk and safety: while professionals may focus on physical harm to the person and others, self-neglect and physical health, the individual may be more concerned about loss of freedom, loss of face, loss of friends, job, college place ... A safety plan must seek to mitigate risks from everyone's perspective. For example, John was compulsorily detained with suspected drug-induced psychosis. Staff were concerned about the safety of others and the risk of his getting access to drugs, therefore he was not allowed to leave the ward and his girlfriend was banned because it was suspected she might bring him drugs. This led to John repeatedly trying to abscond and very poor relationships between John and the ward staff. Another way?

(continued)

continued . . .

> *John's primary concerns were that he would lose his girlfriend and his college place. A safety plan might be drawn up between the three of them addressing the concerns of both the staff and John. All could agree that the aim should be to enable John to return to his girlfriend and his college course as soon as possible. John's girlfriend might be allowed to visit him, initially on the ward, on condition that she did not bring in drugs. Initially, a urine test might be used to check that he had not used drugs. John might be assisted to contact his college and say that he was unwell – maybe ask for some of the work to be sent to him on the ward via his girlfriend so he would not get too far behind. As soon as possible he might start attending his course from the ward before going home to his girlfriend.*

A recovery-focused **safety plan** needs to:

- address risks and concerns from everyone's perspective;
- be explicitly directed towards helping the person to take back control themselves and do the things they value; and
- use all the resources available including the expertise of the individual and those who are close to them.

Individuals and those close to them often know what upsets them, when something is wrong and what helps the person to feel calm and safe. Using this intelligence increases safety. A person (and their relatives as appropriate) might routinely be asked what tends to make them feel upset/angry/unsafe and what helps to mitigate this: this information can then form part of the person's safety plan.

Case study

Julian was in a high dependency forensic unit. From time to time he became very distressed and staff felt it was sometimes necessary to place him in seclusion: often this required restraint, but Julian hated being touched by staff. Therefore, it was agreed that staff would initially ask him to go to seclusion without touching/restraining him: although he continued to shout when asked, he did go voluntarily meaning less risk of physical harm (to staff or Julian) and improved relationships.

It must be remembered that trust is a two-way street: staff cannot expect those using services to trust and respect them unless they show some measure of trust and respect towards the person. If people are to regain personal control then responsibility for safety needs to be shared from the start and gradually handed back to the person. Even if someone is very distressed, some sharing of responsibility may be possible. For example, if someone is on 15 minute observations, consideration might be given to what the person can do if they feel distressed or unsafe between these times (e.g. listen to the radio, go and talk to another resident or member of staff).

Such sharing of responsibility can increase safety.

> ### Case study
>
> *Riya was a long-term resident in a 'challenging behaviour' unit. Every couple of days she became very distressed and a familiar pattern developed: she would become abusive and threaten/hit out at others, then staff would restrain and medicate her after which she would calm down. In discussion with Riya, safety was increased by giving her an increased measure of control and sharing responsibility for safety: it was agreed that when she started to feel angry and upset she come and ask staff for prn medication and they would give it to her when she requested it. This simple agreement reduced violent incidents considerably.*

Such collaborative approaches to safety are not easy. There will be times when people are not willing or able to engage in discussion but, as well as explaining how we are doing things, we can still listen to, take seriously and record their side of the story. It is only by doing this that we can build up the mutual understanding that forms the basis of collaborative working. This brings back the central theme of this chapter which is that only by understanding the person in their own personal, social, cultural and political context and valuing them as individuals can we engage in effective recovery-focused relationships, which inspire hope, give people a sense of control and enable them to participate in opportunities within their own life. Whilst these examples have been in the context of inpatient mental health, these principles and approaches can equally be applied across all health conditions, services and settings.

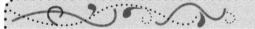

Chapter summary

This chapter has explored the role of the mental health nurse in promoting recovery within hospitals and secure units, for service users who are away from their own homes and surroundings. The importance of allowing service user participation in their own care, even when the options available to them for choice are very limited, has been raised. It looks at ways of redefining risk and safety planning.

The chapter acknowledges there are complexities in developing recovery approaches in inpatient mental health settings, but it has used examples to explore ways of inspiring hope, and offering choice and control as well as opportunities to participate.

Activity: Brief outline answer

Activity 7.2: Communication (page 101)

	Encouraging	**Neutral**	**Discouraging**	**Stigmatising**
Statement	That's great! Well done!	He has two children who he visits regularly	He will never be able to do that!	Drug addicts are always unreliable

(continued)

(continued)

	Encouraging	Neutral	Discouraging	Stigmatising
Description	A man who is working towards turning his life around	A 36-year-old gentleman	He has not achieved much in his life	He is a drug addict
Open question	What can I do to help you?	How are you?	What could he achieve given his unreliability?	Well, what do you expect from him?
Closed question	Would you like me to help you?	Do you have children?	You have tried this before and failed, haven't you?	You never learn, do you?

Further reading

Boardman, J. and Roberts, G. (2014) *Risk, safety and recovery.* ImROC Briefing Paper, London: Centre for Mental Health and Mental Health Network, NHS Confederation. www.imroc.org/media/publications/

Perkins, R. and Repper, J. (2016) Recovery vs risk? From managing risk to the co-production of safety and opportunity. *Mental Health and Social Inclusion*, 20 (2), 101–9.

Useful website

www.imroc.org Implementing Recovery through Organisational Change (ImROC).

Glossary

Alzheimer's disease: the most common form of dementia characterised by progressive memory loss, confusion, disorientation, and problems with decision-making and reasoning skills.

amygdala: the structure in the brain thought to be linked to both fear responses and pleasure.

auditory hallucinations: an abnormal experience resulting from an underlying biological dysfunction which requires medical care and treatment.

biomedical model: conceptualises health and illness biologically.

biopsychosocial model: identifies how psychological and social experiences combine with biological factors to affect the course of illness and health outcomes.

cognitive behavioural therapy: a talking therapy that supports coping and problem-solving by changing the way people think and behave.

community: not only geographical community where people live but:

- communities of identification: people who the person sees as being like them for example, helping someone to access a particular faith community or lesbian/gay community;
- communities of interest: people who share interests with the person, for example, political parties, sporting or arts activities;
- e-communities and opportunities: the internet contains a wealth of information and possibilities for contact, and e-exclusion simply compounds the exclusion that is so often a consequence of mental health challenges thus rendering the person further isolated and alone;
- peer communities: peer-led groups and organisations as well as individuals within the person's network who share similar challenges.

Community Treatment Orders (CTO): set out the terms under which a person must accept medication and therapy, counselling, management, rehabilitation and other services while living in the community.

complete recovery: where an individual returns to their level of functioning before they experienced mental ill health, often implying that the person has been 'cured' or *recovered*.

dopamine: a neurotransmitter involved in controlling the brain's reward and pleasure centres.

frontal cortex: the frontal part of the brain which is thought to control motor function, problem-solving, spontaneity, memory, language, initiation, judgement, impulse control, and social and sexual behavior.

hippocampus: the structure in the brain thought to be at the centre of emotion, memory and the autonomic nervous system.

holism: the view that sees our health being influenced by interconnected social factors, physical, psychological, emotional and spiritual dimensions of self.

hope: goal-directed thinking in which the person is able to find routes to desired goals and is motivated to use those routes.

institutionalisation: the dehumanising, psychological and mental health effects of living for a long time in an institution where the demands on the institution take precedence over the needs of the individual.

Johari window: a technique for understanding ourselves that we, and others, may or may not see.

labelling: the judgements, often negative, made by a community about an individual/individuals whose behaviour violates social norms.

mental wellbeing: comprises our subjective mental health, happiness, hope and optimism and life satisfaction, positive psychological functioning, resilience to adversity, autonomy and a sense of control over one's life, self-awareness and acceptance, and supportive and interpersonal relationships.

person-centred approach: based on the work of Carl Rogers, this approach puts the patient/service user at the heart of care processes and stresses the importance of democratising decision-making and the human experience of health care, as well as evidence-based treatments and interventions.

personal values: personal standards and moral judgements about what is important in life.

recovery: a personal, unique process of changing one's attitudes, values, feelings, goals, skills and/or roles with the aim of developing a satisfying, hopeful and contributing life even with limitations caused by mental health problems.

resilience: the ability to bounce back or positively adapt in the face of significant adversity or risk.

responsible clinician: the mental health professional who has overall responsibility for the care and treatment of service users being assessed and treated under the Mental Health Act.

safety plan: co-created risk management plans which address risks and concerns from everyone's perspective; are explicitly directed towards helping the person to take back control themselves and do the things they value; and use all the resources available including the expertise of the individual and those who are close to them.

schizophrenia: a mental health condition characterised by hallucinations, delusions, disorganised thoughts and behaviour changes.

self-efficacy: the belief in one's ability and capabilities when required by any given situation.

social exclusion: the exclusion or expulsion of individuals from the prevailing social system and its rights and privileges.

social inclusion: the active involvement of individuals in their communities and society as citizens which bestows benefits and rights.

social recovery: emphasises social support, realistic planning, significant working relationships, encouragement, appropriate treatment, choice and self-management.

spoiled identity: an identity that causes a person to experience stigma.

Stress Vulnerability Model: the model developed by Zubin and Spring (1977) which identifies how the mental health and wellbeing of people diagnosed with schizophrenia and their ability to cope at times of adversity is influenced by inherited genetic background and life experiences and external stressors (such as significant life events like deaths, divorce, financial problems and so on).

therapeutic relationship: a supportive, person-centred alliance between a service user and health care professional.

Tidal Model: based on the work of Barker (2001); places interpersonal relations at the heart of nursing practice.

variables: any factor that can be controlled, changed or measured.

References

Ackerman, S.J. and Hilsenroth, M.J. (2003) A review of therapist characteristics and techniques positively impacting on the therapeutic alliance. *Clinical Psychology Review*, 23, 1–33.

Allen, S. (2010) *Our stories: Moving on. Recovery and well-being.* London: South West London and St. George's Mental Health NHS Trust.

American Psychiatric Association (APA) (2013) *Diagnostic and statistical manual of mental disorders* (5th edn). Arlington, VA: American Psychiatric Publishing.

Anthony, W.A. (1993) Recovery from mental illness: The guiding vision of the mental health system in the 1990s. *Psychosocial Rehabilitation Journal*, 16, 11–23.

Appleby, L., Mortensen, P.B., Dunn, G. and Hiroeh, U. (2001) Death by homicide, suicide, and other unnatural causes in people with mental illness: a population-based study. *The Lancet*, 358, 2110–12.

Aslan, M. and Smith, M. (2012) Promoting health and social inclusion. In Tee, S., Brown, J. and Carpenter, D. (eds) *Handbook of mental health nursing.* London: Hodder Arnold, pp187–207.

Barker, P. (2001) The Tidal Model: developing an empowering, person-centred approach to recovery within psychiatric and mental health nursing. *Journal of Psychiatric and Mental Health Nursing*, 8 (3), 233–40.

Barker, P. (2004) *Assessment in psychiatric and mental health nursing* (2nd edn). Cheltenham: Nelson Thornes.

Barker, P. and Buchanan-Barker, P. (2005) *The Tidal Model: A guide for mental health professionals.* London and New York: Brunner Routledge.

Barker, P. and Buchanan-Barker, P. (2011) Myth of mental health nursing and the challenge of recovery. *International Journal of Mental Health Nursing*, 20, 337–44.

Barker, P., Jackson, S. and Stevenson, C. (1999) What are psychiatric nurses needed for? Developing a theory of essential nursing practice. *Journal of Psychiatric and Mental Health Nursing*, 6, 273–82.

Barker, P., Stevenson, C. and Leamy, M. (2000) The philosophy of empowerment. *Mental Health Nursing*, 20 (9), 8–12.

Beck, J.S. (2011) *Cognitive behavior therapy: Basics and beyond* (2nd edn). London: The Guilford Press.

Bentall, R. (2003) *Madness explained: Psychosis and human nature.* London: Penguin.

Berry, C., Hayward, M. and Porter, A. (2008) Evaluating socially inclusive practice: Part one – a tool for mental health services. *Journal of Mental Health Training, Education and Practice*, 3 (4), 31–41.

Berry, C., Gerry, L., Hayward, M. and Chandler, R. (2010) Expectations and illusions: A position paper on the relationship between mental health practitioners and social exclusion. *Journal of Psychiatric and Mental Health Nursing*, 17 (5), 411–21.

Better Regulation Commission (2006) *Risk responsibility and regulation: Whose risk is it anyway?* London: Better Regulation Commission.

Boardman, J. and Roberts, G. (2014) *Risk, safety and recovery.* ImROC Briefing Paper, London: Centre for Mental Health and Mental Health Network, NHS Confederation. www.imroc.org/media/publications/

Bowers, L., Alexander, J., Bilgion, H., Botgha, M., Dack, C., James, K., Jarrett, M., Jeffrey, D., Nijman, H., Owili, J.A., Papadopoulos, C., Ross, J., Wright, S. and Stewart, D. (2014) Safewards: The empirical basis of the model and a critical appraisal. *Journal of Psychiatric and Mental Health Nursing*, 21 (4), 354–64.

Brittan, A. and Maynard, M. (1984) *Sexism, racism and oppression.* New York: Basil Blackwell.

Brown, M. (2004) *Coping with depression after traumatic brain injury.* www.biausa.org/_literature_43189/depression_and_brain_injury.

Burns, T., Rugkasa, J., Molodynski, A., Dawson, J., Yeeles, K., Vazquez-Montes, M., et al. (2013) Community treatment orders for patients with psychosis (OCTET): A randomised controlled trial. *Lancet*, 81 (9878), 1627–33.

Cahill, J. (2009) A combined review of: Collective biography and the legacy of Hildegard Peplau, Annie Altschul and Eileen Skellern; the origins of mental health nursing and its relevance to the current crisis in psychiatry; Mental health content of comprehensive pre-registration nursing curricula in Australia and Childhood abuse and psychosis; a critical review of the literature. *Journal of Research in Nursing*, 14, 549.

Cameron, D., Kapur, R. and Campbell, P. (2005) Releasing the therapeutic potential of the psychiatric nurse: A human relations perspective of the nurse–patient relationship. *Journal of Psychiatric and Mental Health Nursing*, 12, 64–74.

Campbell, P. (2005) From Little Acorns: The mental health service user movement. In *Beyond the water towers.* London: Sainsbury Centre for Mental Health.

Care Quality Commission (2014) *Monitoring the Mental Health Act in 2013/14.* www.cqc.org.uk/sites/default/files/monitoring_the_mha_2013-14_report_web_0303.pdf.pdf.

Care Services Improvement Partnership (2007) *Strengthening the involvement of people with dementia.* London: CSIP Older People's Mental Health Programme.

Chadwick, P.K. (1997) *Schizophrenia: The positive perspective. In search of dignity for schizophrenic people.* London: Routledge.

Cleary, M. (2004) The realities of mental health nursing in acute inpatient environments. *International Journal of Mental Health Nursing*, 13, 53–60.

Clifton, A., Repper, J., Banks, D. and Remnant, J. (2013) Co-producing social inclusion: The structure/agency conundrum. *Journal of Psychiatric and Mental Health Nursing*, 20, 514–24.

Collins, P.H. (1986) Learning from the outsider within: The sociological significance of Black feminist thought. *Social Problems.* University of California, ppS14–S32.

Cowman, S., Farelly, M. and Gilheany, P. (2001) An examination of the role and function of psychiatric nurses in clinical practice in Ireland. *Journal of Advanced Nursing*, 34 (6), 745–53.

Cromer-Hayes, M. and Chandley, M. (2015) Recovery in a high secure hospital in England. *Mental Health Practice*, 18 (8), 32–7.

Csikszentmihalyi, M. (1975) *Beyond boredom and anxiety: Experiencing flow in work and play.* San Francisco: Jossey-Bass.

Cutcliffe, J.R. and Koehn, C.V. (2007) Hope and interpersonal psychiatric/mental health nursing: A systematic review of the literature – Part II. *Journal of Psychiatric and Mental Health Nursing*, 14, 141–7.

Daley, S., Newton, D., Slade, M. et al (2013) Development of a framework for recovery for older people with mental disorder. *International Journal of Geriatric Psychiatry*, 28, 522–9.

Danzinger, K. (1976) *Interpersonal communication.* Oxford: Pergamon Press.

De Beauvoir, S. (1949) *The second sex.* Paris: Gallimard.

Deegan, P.E. (1988) Recovery: The lived experience of rehabilitation. *Psychosocial Rehabilitation Journal*, 9 (4), 11–19.

Deegan, P. (1992) The Independent Living Movement and people with psychiatric disabilities: Taking back control over our lives. *Psychosocial Rehabilitation Journal*, 15 (3), 3–19.

Deegan, P. (1993) Recovering our sense of value after being labelled mentally ill. *Journal of Psychosocial Nursing and Mental Health Services*, 31, 7–11.

Deegan, P. (1996) 'There's a person in here': *The Sixth Annual Mental Health Services Conference of Australia and New Zealand.* Brisbane, Australia, 16 September 1996.

Deegan, P.E. (2007) The lived experience of using psychiatric medication in the recovery process and a shared decision-making program to support it. *Psychiatric Rehabilitation Journal*, 31 (1), 62–9.

Deegan, P. and Drake, R. (2006) Shared decision making and medication management in the recovery process. *Psychiatric Services*, 57, 1636–9.

Deegan, P., Rapp, C., Holter, M. and Reifer, M. (2008) A program to support shared decision making in an outpatient psychiatric medication clinic. *Psychiatric Services*, 59, 603–5.

Department of Health (DH) (2004) *The Ten Essential Shared Capabilities: A Framework for the Whole of the Mental Health Workforce.* http://webarchive.nationalarchives.gov.uk/20130107105354/http://www.dh.gov.uk/prod_consum_dh/groups/dh_digitalassets/@dh/@en/documents/digitalasset/dh_4087170.pdf.

Department of Health (DH) (2006a) *Reviewing the care programme approach.* London: Department of Health.

Department of Health (DH) (2006b) *From values to action: The Chief Nursing Officer's review of mental health nursing.* http://webarchive.nationalarchives.gov.uk/+/www.dh.gov.uk/en/Consultations/Closedconsultations/DH_4121787

Department of Health (DH) (2007) *Capabilities for inclusive practice.* https://www2.rcn.org.uk/__data/assets/pdf_file/0008/513782/dh-2007-capabilities-for-inclusive-practice.pdf.

Department of Health (DH) (2008) *High quality care for all: NHS next stage review final report.* London: Department of Health.

Department of Health (DH) (2010) *Equity and excellence: Liberating the NHS*. www.gov.uk/government/uploads/system/uploads/attachment_data/file/213823/dh_117794.pdf

Department of Health (DH) (2011) *No health without mental health: A cross government mental health outcomes strategy for people of all ages*. www.gov.uk/government/uploads/system/uploads/attachment_data/file/213761/dh_124058.pdf.

Department of Health (DH) (2012) *Transforming care: A national response to Winterbourne View Hospital*. London: Department of Health.

Department of Health (DH) (2013) *The NHS Constitution*. www.gov.uk/government/uploads/system/uploads/attachment_data/file/170656/NHS_Constitution.pdf.

Department of Health (DH) (2015) *The NHS Constitution*. www.gov.uk/government/uploads/system/uploads/attachment_data/file/480482/NHS_Constitution_WEB.pdf.

Department of Health and Concordat Signatories (2014) *Mental Health Crisis Care Concordat: Improving outcomes for people experiencing mental health crisis*. www.gov.uk/government/uploads/system/uploads/attachment_data/file/281242/36353_Mental_Health_Crisis_accessible.pdf

Diener, E., Emmons, R.A., Larsen, R.J. and Giffin, S. (1985) The Satisfaction with Life Scale. *Journal of Personality Assessment*, 49, 1, 71–5.

Drennan, G. et al. (2014) *Making recovery a reality in mental health settings*. London: Centre for Mental Health and Mental Health Network.

Egan, G. (1994) *The skilled helper* (5th edn). Belmont, CA: Brooks/Cole Publishing Company.

Egan, G. (2010) *The skilled helper* (9th edn). California: Pacific Grove.

Engel, G. (1977) The need for a new medical model. *Science*, 196, 129–36.

Forchuk, C. and Reynolds, W. (2001) Clients' reflections on relationships with nurses: Comparisons from Canada and Scotland. *Journal of Psychiatric and Mental Health Nursing*, 8, 45–51.

Francis, R. (Chair) (2013) *Report of the Mid Staffordshire NHS Foundation Trust Public Inquiry*. London: The Stationery Office.

Friedli, L. (2009) *Mental health, resilience and inequalities*. Denmark: World Health Organization Europe.

Gilburt, H., Rose, D. and Slade, M. (2008) The importance of relationships in mental health care: A qualitative study of service users' experiences of psychiatric hospital admission in the UK. *BMC Health Services Research*, 8, 92.

Goffman, E. (1963) *Stigma: Notes on the management of spoiled identity*. New York: Simon and Schuster.

Griffiths, K.M., Carron-Arthur, B., Parsons, A. and Reid, R. (2014) Effectiveness of programs for reducing the stigma associated with mental disorders: A meta-analysis of randomized controlled trials. *World Psychiatry*, 13 (2), 161–75.

Gureje, O. (2007) Psychiatric aspects of pain. *Current Opinion in Psychiatry*, 20, 42–6.

Hannigan, B. and Burnard, P. (2000) Nursing, politics and policy: A response to Clifford. *Nurse Education Today*, 20 (7), 519–23.

Henderson, C., Flood, C., Leese, M., Thornicroft, G., Sutherby, K. and Szmukler, G. (2004) Effect of joint crisis plans on use of compulsory treatment in psychiatry: Single blind randomised controlled trial. *BMJ*, 329 (7458), 136.

References

Hill, L., Roberts, G., Wildgoose, J., Perkins, R. and Hahn, S. (2010) Recovery and person-centred care in dementia: Common purpose, common practice? *Advances in Psychiatric Treatment*, 16, 288–98.

House, J.S., Landis, K.R. and Umberson, D. (1988) Social relationships and health. *Science*, 241: 540–5.

Jacobson, N. and Greenley, D. (2001) What is recovery? A conceptual model and explication. *Psychiatric Services*, 52 (4), 482–5.

Jenkins, R., Meltzer, H., Jones, P.B., Brugha, T., Bebbington, P., Farrell, M., Crepaz-Keay, D. and Knapp, M. (2008) *Foresight mental capital and wellbeing project. Mental health: Future challenges*. London: The Government Office for Science.

Keeling, J.L. and McQuarrie, C. (2014) Promoting mental health and wellbeing in practice. *Mental Health Practice*, 17 (5), 26–8.

Kisely, S.R., Campbell, L.A. and Preston, N.J. (2011) Compulsory community and involuntary outpatient treatment for people with severe mental disorders. *Cochrane Database of Systematic Reviews*, 2, CD004408.

Kring, A., Johnson, S., Davison, G. and Neale, J. (2010) *Abnormal Psychology* (11th edn). Hoboken, NJ: Wiley.

Kylmä, J., Juvakka, T., Nikkonen, M., Korhonen, T. and Isohanni, M. (2006) Hope and schizophrenia: An integrative review. *Journal of Psychiatric and Mental Health Nursing*, 13, 651–64.

Lambert, M.J. and Barley, D.E. (2002) Research summary on the therapeutic relationship and psychotherapeutic outcome. In Norcross, J. (ed.) *Psychotherapy relationships that work: Therapist responsibility and contribution to patients*. Oxford: Oxford University Press.

Langan, J. and Lindow, V. (2004) *Living with risk: Mental health service user involvement in risk assessment and management*. Bristol: Policy Press.

Leamy, M., Bird, V., Le Boutillier, C., Williams, J. and Slade, M. (2011) Conceptual framework for personal recovery in mental health: Systematic review and narrative synthesis. *British Journal of Psychiatry*, 199 (6), 445–52.

Leiter, M.P. and Maslach, C. (2009) Nurse turnover: The mediating role of burnout. *Journal of Nursing Management*, 17, 331–9.

Leitner, M. and Barr, W. (2011) Understanding and managing self-harm in mental health services. In Whittington, R. and Logan, C. (eds) *Self-harm and violence: Towards best practice in managing risk in mental health services*. Chichester: Wiley-Blackwell, pp. 55–78.

Levitas, R., Pantazis, C., Fahmy, E., Gordon, D., Lloyd, E. and Patsios, D. (2007) *The multi-dimensional analysis of social exclusion*. http://roar.uel.ac.uk/1781/1/multidimensional.pdf.

Logan, C., Nedopil, N. and Wolf, T. (2011) Guidelines and standards for managing risk in mental health services. In Whittington, R. and Logan, C. (eds) *Self-harm and violence: Towards best practice in managing risk in mental health services*. Chichester: Wiley-Blackwell, pp. 145–62.

Lorde, A. (1984) *Sister outsider*. California: Crossing Press.

Lyubomirsky, S. and Lepper, H. (1999) A measure of subjective happiness: Preliminary reliability and construct validation. *Social Indicators Research*, 46, 137–55.

Margereson, C. and Trenoweth, S. (2010) Epidemiology and aetiology of long-term conditions. In Margereson, C. and Trenoweth, S. (eds) *Developing holistic care for long-term conditions*. London: Routledge.

Marmot, M. (2010) *Fairer society, healthy lives: The Marmot Review executive summary*. www.instituteofhealthequity. org/projects/fair-society-healthy-lives-the-marmot-review.

Matthews, J. (2008) The meaning of recovery. In Lynch, J. and Trenoweth, S. (eds) *Contemporary issues in mental health nursing*. Chichester, Wiley.

Mental Health Act Commission (2009) Coercion and consent. www.cqc.org.uk/sites/default/files/ documents/mhac_biennial_report_0709_final.pdf.

Mental Health Foundation (MHF) (2006) *Feeding minds: The impact of food on mental health*. www.mental health.org.uk/campaigns/food-and-mental-health/

Mental Health Foundation (MHF) (2012) *Service user's experiences of recovery under the 2008 Care Programme Approach*. www.mentalhealth.org.uk/content/assets/PDF/publications/CPA_exec_summary. pdf.

Mental Health Taskforce (2016) *The five year forward view for mental health*. www.england.nhs.uk/wp-content/ uploads/2016/02/Mental-Health-Taskforce-FYFV-final.pdf.

Miller, W.R. and Rollnick, S. (1991) *Motivational interviewing: Preparing people to change addictive behavior.* New York: Guilford Press.

Mind (2011) *Listening to experience.* www.mind.org.uk/media/211306/listening_to_experience_web.pdf

Morgan, C., Burns, T., Fitzpatrick, R., Pinfold, V. and Priebe, S. (2007) Social exclusion and mental health: Conceptual and methodological review. *British Journal of Psychiatry*, 191, 477–83.

Morgan, P. and Lawson, J. (2015) Developing guidelines for sharing lived experience of staff in health and social care. *Mental Health and Social Inclusion*, 19 (2), 78–86.

Morrisey, J. and Callaghan, P. (2011) *Communication skills for mental health nurses: An introduction*. London: McGraw Hill Education.

National Institute for Health and Care Excellence (NICE) (2009) *Depression in adults: Recognition and management*. www.nice.org.uk/guidance/cg90?unlid=292261183201624213554.

National Institute for Health and Care Excellence (NICE) (2012) *Patient experience in adult NHS services*. www.nice.org.uk/guidance/cg138.

National Institute for Mental Health in England (NIMHE) (2005) *NIMHE guiding statement on recovery*. https://manchester.rl.talis.com/items/1462D9CA-3228-11C7-CA3F-429526E1FC79.html.

Nursing and Midwifery Council (NMC) (2010) *Standards for pre-registration nursing education*. www.nmc.org. uk/globalassets/sitedocuments/nmc-publications/standards-for-pre-registration-nursing-education-16082010.pdf

Nursing and Midwifery Council (NMC) (2015) *The Code: Professional standards of practice and behaviour for nurses and midwives.* www.nmc.org.uk/globalassets/sitedocuments/nmc-publications/revised-new-nmc-code.pdf

Office of the Deputy Prime Minister (ODPM) (2004) *Mental health and social exclusion: Social exclusion report.* London: TSO.

O'Hagan, M. (1996) Two accounts of mental distress. In Read, J. and Reynolds, J. (eds) *Speaking our minds.* London: Macmillan/Open University.

References

O'Hagan, M. (2014) *Madness made me.* Wellington, New Zealand: Open Books.

Oliver, M. (2004) If I had a hammer: The social model in action. In Swain, J., French, S., Barnes, C. and Thomas, C. (eds) *Disabling barriers: Enabling environments.* London: Sage.

Olsen, D.P. (1997) When the patient causes the problem: The effect of patient responsibility on the nurse–patient relationship. *Journal of Advanced Nursing,* 26, 515–22.

Onken, S.J., Dumont, J.M., Ridgeway, P., et al. (2002) *Mental health recovery: What helps and what hinders?* Alexandria, VA: National Technical Assistance Center for State Mental Health Planning (NTAC), National Association for State Mental Health Program Directors (NASMHPD).

Park, N., Peterson, C. and Seligman, M. (2004) Strengths of character and well-being. *Journal of Social and Clinical Psychology,* 23 (5), 603–19.

Patel, V. (2015) Addressing social injustice: A key public mental health strategy. *World Psychiatry,* 14 (1), 43–4.

Peck, E. and Norman, I. (1999) Working together in adult community mental health services: Exploring inter-professional role relations. *Journal of Mental Health,* 8 (3), 231–42.

Peplau, H. (1952) *Interpersonal relations in nursing.* London: Macmillan.

Perkins, R. (2012) UK mental health policy development: An alternative view. In Phillips, P., Sandford, T. and Johnston, C. (eds) *Working in mental health: Practice and policy in a changing environment.* Oxford: Routledge.

Perkins, R. (2013) *Surviving and thriving at work.* London: Disability Rights UK.

Perkins, R. and Goddard, K. (2008) Sharing responsibility for risk and risk-taking. *Module 5 of Realising recovery: A national framework for learning and training in recovery focused practice.* NHS Education for Scotland. www.nes.scot.nhs.uk/education-and-training/by-theme-initiative/mental-health-and-learning-disabilities/publication.

Perkins, R. and Repper, J. (2015) Recovery is possible for everyone? *Mental Health and Social Inclusion,* 19 (2), 57–60.

Perkins, R. and Repper, J. (2016) Recovery versus risk? From managing risk to the co-production of safety and opportunity. *Mental Health and Social Inclusion,* 20 (2), 101–9.

Perna, R. et al. (2003) Traumatic brain injury: Depression, neurogenesis and medication management. *Journal of Head Trauma Rehabilitation,* 18 (2), 201–3.

Pescosolido, B.A. (2013) The public stigma of mental illness: What do we think; what do we know; what can we prove? *Journal of Health and Social Behavior,* 54 (1), 1–21.

Pettie, D. and Triolo, A.M. (1999) Illness as evolution: The search for identity and meaning in the recovery process. *Psychiatric Rehabilitation Journal,* 22 (3), 255.

Pratt, R. and Wilkinson, H. (2001) Tell me the truth: The effect of being told the diagnosis of dementia from the perspective of the person with dementia. London: Mental Health Foundation.

Ralph, R.O. (2000) *Review of recovery literature: A synthesis of a sample of recovery literature.* Alexandria, VA: National Technical Assistance Center for State Mental Health Planning (NTAC), National Association for State Mental Health Program Directors (NASMHPD).

Repper, J. and Perkins, R. (2003) *Social inclusion and recovery: A model for mental health practice.* Edinburgh: Bailliere Tindall.

Repper, J. and Perkins, R. (2012) Recovery: A journey of discovery for individuals and services. In Phillips, P., Sandford, T. and Johnston, C. (eds) *Working in mental health: Practice and policy in a challenging environment.* Oxford: Routledge.

Repper, J., Aldridge, B., Gilfoyle, S., Gillard, S., Perkins, R. and Rennison, J. (2013a) *Peer support workers: Theory and practice.* ImROC briefing paper. London: ImROC, NHS Confederation Mental Health Network/ Centre for Mental Health, London. www.imroc.org/media/publications/

Repper, J., Aldridge, B., Gilfoyle, S., Gillard, S., Perkins, R. and Rennison, J. (2013b) *Peer support workers: A practical guide to implementation.* ImROC briefing paper. London: ImROC, NHS Confederation Mental Health Network/Centre for Mental Health, London. www.imroc.org/media/publications/

Ridgeway, P. (2001) Restoring psychiatric disability: Learning from first-person accounts of recovery. *Psychiatric Rehabilitation Journal,* 24 (4), 335–43.

Roberts, G. and Boardman, J. (2014) Becoming a recovery-oriented practitioner. *Advances in Psychiatric Treatment,* 20 (1), 37–47.

Roberts, G., Dorkins, E., Wooldridge, J., et al. (2008) Detained – what's my choice? Part 1: Discussion. *Advances in Psychiatric Treatment,* 14: 172–80.

Robinson, J. (1997) Power, politics and policy analysis in nursing. In Perry, A. (ed.) *Nursing: A knowledge base for practice* (2nd edn). London: Arnold, pp249–81.

Rogers, C.R. (1956) reprinted (1992) The necessary and sufficient conditions of therapeutic personality change. *Journal of Consulting and Clinical Psychology,* 60 (6), 827–32.

Rosenfield, S. (2012) Triple jeopardy? Mental health at the intersection of gender, race and class. *Social Science and Medicine,* 74, 1791–801.

Royal College of Psychiatrists (2008) *Rethinking risk to others in mental health services.* College Report CR 150. London: Royal College of Psychiatrists.

Royal College of Psychiatrists (2013) *Whole-person care: From rhetoric to reality. Achieving parity between mental and physical health. Summary.* www.rcpsych.ac.uk/pdf/OP88summary.pdf.

Royal College of Psychiatrists Social Inclusion Scoping Group (2009) *Position Statement. Mental health and social inclusion: Making psychiatry and mental health services fit for the 21st century.* www.rcpsych.ac.uk/pdf/ PS01_2009x.pdf.

Ryan, S.F. (2015) *Nurse practitioners and political engagement: Findings from a nurse practitioner advanced practice focus group and national online survey.* http://anp-foundation.org/wp-content/uploads/2015/04/Nurse_ Practitioners_and_Political_Engagement_Report.pdf.

Ryff, C. (1989). Happiness is everything, or is it? Explorations on the meaning of psychological well-being. *Journal of Personality and Social Psychology,* 57, 1069–81.

Ryff, C. and Keyes, C. (1995) The structure of psychological well-being revisited. *Journal of Personality and Social Psychology,* 69, 719–27.

Safewards (2016) *Know each other.* http://www.safewards.net/interventions/know-each-other

Sayce, L. (2001) Social inclusion and mental health. *The Psychiatrist*, 25 (4), 121–3.

Schein, E.H. (2013) *Humble inquiry: The gentle are to asking instead of telling*. San Francisco: Berrett-Koehler.

Scott-Moncrieff, L., Briscoe, J. and Daniels, G. (2009) *An independent investigation into the care and treatment of Daniel Gonzales*. NHS South East Coast (formerly Surrey and Sussex SHA) and Surrey County Council.

Seligman, M. (2002) *Authentic happiness*. London: Nicholas Brearley Publishing.

Sells, D., Borg, M., Marin, I., et al. (2006) Arenas of recovery for persons with severe mental illness. *American Journal of Psychiatry and Rehabilitation*, 9, 3–16.

Shepherd, G., Boardman, J. and Slade, M. (2008) *Making recovery a reality*. London: Sainsbury Centre for Mental Health.

Shepherd, G., Boardman, J., Rinaldi, M. and Roberts, G. (2014) *Supporting recovery in mental health services. Quality and outcomes: Implementing recovery through organisational change*. London: Sainsbury Centre for Mental Health.

Slade, M. (2009a) *Personal recovery and mental illness: A guide for mental health professionals*. Cambridge: Cambridge University Press.

Slade, M. (2009b) *100 ways to support recovery*. London: Rethink.

Slade, M., Amering, M., Farkas, M., Hamilton, B., O'Hagan, M., Panther, G., Perkins, R., Shepherd, G., Tse, S. and Whitley, R. (2014) Uses and abuses of recovery: Implementing recovery-oriented practices in mental health systems. *World Psychiatry* 13 (1), 12–20.

Smith, B.T., Padgett, D.K., Choy-Brown, M. and Henwood, B.F. (2015) Rebuilding lives and identities: The role of place in recovery among persons with complex needs. *Health and Place*, 33, 109–17.

Snyder, R., Lopez, S. and Pedrotti, J. (2011) *Positive psychology: The scientific and practical explorations of human strengths* (2nd edn). Thousand Oaks, CA: Sage Publications.

Social Care Institute for Excellence (2006) *Assessing the mental health needs of older people*. London: Social Care Institute for Excellence.

Stewart-Brown, S. and Janmohamed, K. (2008) *Warwick-Edinburgh Mental Well-being Scale (WEMWBS) User Guide Version 1*. www.mentalhealthpromotion.net/resources/user-guide.pdf

Sully, P. and Dalas, J. (2005) *Essential communication skills for nursing*. Oxford: Elsevier Health Sciences.

Swinton, J. (2001) *Spirituality and mental health care: Rediscovering a forgotten dimension*. London: Jessica Kingsley.

Thurgood, M. (2009) Engaging clients in their care and treatment. In Norman, I. and Ryrie, I. (eds) *The art and science of mental health nursing: A textbook of principle and practice* (2nd edn). Maidenhead: Open University Press.

Timmermans, S. and Mauck, A. (2005) The promises and pitfalls of evidence-based medicine. *Health Affairs*, 24 (1), 18–28.

Tooth, B., Kalyanasundaram, V., Glover, H., et al. (2003) Factors consumers identify as important to recovery from schizophrenia. *Australasian Psychiatry* 11 (1), 70–7.

Traynor, M. (2014) Caring after Francis: Moral failure in nursing reconsidered. *Journal of Research in Nursing,* 19 (7–8), 546–56.

Trenoweth, S. and Larter, A. (2008) Rebuilding lives: A critical look at the contemporary role of the mental health nurse. In Lynch, J.E. and Trenoweth, S. (eds) *Contemporary Issues in Mental Health Nursing.* Chichester: Wiley.

Umphrey, L.R. and Sherblom, J.C. (2014) The relationship of hope to self-compassion, relational social skill, communication apprehension, and life satisfaction. *International Journal of Wellbeing,* 4 (2), 1–18.

United Nations (2006) UN Convention on the Rights of Persons with Disabilities. www.un.org/disabilities/convention/conventionfull.shtml.

US Department of Health and Human Services, Substance Abuse and Mental Health Services Administration (2011) *Shared decision-making in mental health care practice.* Rockville, MD: SAMHSA.

Van Bogaert, P., Kowalski, C., Mace Weeks, S., Van Heusden, D. and Clarke, S.P. (2013) The relationship between nurse practice environment, nurse work characteristics, burnout and job outcome and quality of care: A cross sectional study. *International Journal of Nursing Studies,* 50, 1667–77.

Viney, L.L. (1986) Expression of positive emotion by people who are physically ill: Is it evidence of defending or coping? In Gottschalk, L.A., Lolas, F. and Viney, L.L. (eds) *Content analysis of verbal behaviour: Significance in clinical medicine and psychiatry.* Berlin: Springer-Verlag.

Viney, L.L. and Henry, R.M. (2002) Evaluating personal construct and psychodynamic group work with adolescent offenders and nonoffenders. In Neimeyer, R.A. and Neimeyer, G.J. (eds) *Advances in personal construct psychology: New directions and perspectives.* Westport, CT: Praeger.

Warner, R. (1985) *Recovery from schizophrenia: Psychiatry and political economy.* London: Routledge and Kegan Paul.

Warner, R. (2009) Recovery from schizophrenia and the recovery model. *Current Opinions in Psychiatry,* 22 (4), 374–80.

Watkins, P. (2001) *Mental health nursing: The art of compassionate care.* Edinburgh: Butterworth Heinemann.

Watkins, P. (2009) *Compassionate care: A guide for mental health practitioners.* London: Elsevier.

Westbrook, M.T. (1976) Positive affect: A method of content analysis for verbal samples. *Journal of Consulting and Clinical Psychology,* 44 (5), 715–19.

Westbrook, M.T. and Viney, L.L. (1980) Scales for measuring people's perception of themselves as origins and pawns. *Journal of Personality Assessment,* 44 (2), 167–74.

Wood, R. and Bandura, A. (1989) Impact of conceptions of ability on self-regulatory mechanisms and complex decision making. *Journal of Personality and Social Psychology,* 56, 407–15.

Woodward, B., Smart, D. and Benavides-Vaello, S. (2016) Modifiable factors that support political participation by nurses. *Journal of Professional Nursing,* 32 (1), 54–61.

World Health Organization (WHO) (1946) *Preamble to the Constitution of the World Health Organization as adopted by the International Health Conference,* New York, 19–22 June, 1946; signed on 22 July 1946 by the representatives of 61 States (Official Records of the World Health Organization, no. 2, p. 100) and entered into force on 7 April 1948.

World Health Organization (WHO) (2007a) *International Classification of Diseases (ICD) 10th edn: Version 2015.* http://apps.who.int/classifications/icd10/browse/2015/en

World Health Organization (WHO) (2007b) *Mental health: Strengthening our response [online]. Fact sheet N°220.* Media Centre, WHO. www.who.int/mediacentre/factsheets/fs220/en/index.html.

Wright, N. and Stickley, T. (2013) Concepts of social inclusion, exclusion and mental health: A review of the international literature. *Journal of Psychiatric and Mental Health Nursing,* 20, 71–81.

Zubin, J. and Spring, B. (1977) Vulnerability: A new view of schizophrenia. *Journal of Abnormal Psychology,* 86 (2), 103–24.

Index